Kids' Club Letters

Kids' Club Letters

Narrative Tools for Stimulating Process and Dialogue in Therapy Groups for Children and Adolescents

Georgia A. DeGangi
Marc A. Nemiroff

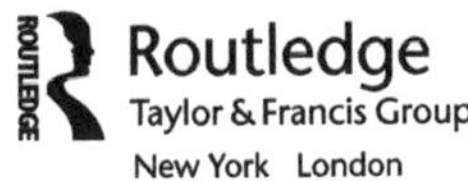

Routledge
Taylor & Francis Group
New York London

Routledge
Taylor & Francis Group
711 Third Avenue
New York, NY 10017

Routledge
Taylor & Francis Group
27 Church Road
Hove, East Sussex BN3 2FA

Routledge is an imprint of Taylor & Francis Group, an Informa business

International Standard Book Number: 978-0-415-99432-3 (Paperback)

Library of Congress Cataloging-in-Publication Data

DeGangi, Georgia A.
Kids' club letters : narrative tools for stimulating process and dialogue in therapy groups for children and adolescents / by Georgia A. DeGangi and Marc A. Nemiroff.
p. ; cm.
Includes bibliographical references and index.
ISBN 978-0-415-99432-3 (pbk. : alk. paper)
1. Group psychotherapy for children. 2. Narrative therapy. I. Nemiroff, Marc A. II. Title.
[DNLM: 1. Psychotherapy, Group--methods. 2. Adolescent. 3. Child. 4. Correspondence as Topic. 5. Narration. WS 350.2 D317k 2009]

RJ505.G7D44 2009
618.92'89152--dc22 2009009421

Visit the Taylor & Francis Web site at
http://www.taylorandfrancis.com

and the Routledge Web site at
http://www.routledgementalhealth.com

Contents

The Therapeutic Technique: Using the Group as an "Advice Column"

This book, unique in its presentation, is intended for mental health professionals and educators. It provides an innovative approach to group psychotherapy for school-aged children who experience a range of primarily co-existing social, emotional, and constitutional problems. A narrative therapy approach was adapted, taking the form of letters, written by the therapist in the voice of a child asking for advice about interpersonal or emotional problems. The "child" in the letter is asking for guidance from the participants in several different groups of children in group psychotherapy. The letters were written with the goals of helping structure responses within each group, and allowing the young participants to address issues that were specifically relevant to them. The children in these groups experienced difficulties discussing these issues spontaneously, and hence the "Dear Kids' Club" letter format was born. The children did not know that the therapist had written the letters.

The topics for the "Dear Kids' Club" letters were generated after several years of qualitative observations by Dr. DeGangi to determine the kinds of problems that children seek or need help with in a group psychotherapy context. The authors selected the letters for this volume based on how the issues cluster in specific themes, such as identity, competence, stress management, conflict-resolution, mood regulation, and interpersonal effectiveness. The authors have chosen to focus on those letters that elicited the most helpful and interesting individual and group responses. Differences by age, gender, and diagnoses of the children (e.g., Asperger's syndrome, anxiety disorders, attention-deficit disorders, and regulatory disorders) are discussed and demonstrated by the wide range of responses that each letter elicited.

Dr. DeGangi was the author of the letters, as well as the primary therapist in the groups. She is the therapist speaking to the children in the group dialogues that appear verbatim in this book. The "Dear Kids' Club" letters were read to the children participating in the groups. Then their responses were recorded and transcribed. Each group consisted of approximately six children, all of the same gender. There were two co-leaders; however, the therapist responses in this book were those of Dr. DeGangi, who was trained as a clinical psychologist.

Format of the Book

The book is organized into three parts.

Part I: Formation of identity and self-understanding
Part II: Interpersonal effectiveness in the forms of problem-solving, decision-making, leadership skills, and listening and conversational skills
Part III: Mood regulation including identifying and understanding emotions, modulation of affect such as anger, and impulse control

The transcribed dialogues of the different groups of children are unedited and provide rich insights into the differing ways that children perceive and interpret their problems. Further, the therapist's responses, and the ensuing clinical discussions by the authors, demonstrate how clinicians might guide group process to help children clarify, elaborate, and understand the ideas and emotional meanings that may arise within any given group session. Not all groups are featured with each letter. Instead, we selected those group sessions that offer the reader insights into group process. Additionally, the authors speak to each other about the prevailing group process and therapeutic decisions that must be made at critical moments during sessions.

Dr. DeGangi and Dr. Nemiroff have decided, in keeping with the essentially conversational clinical material, to discuss the material in a parallel dialogue of their own. After reading the letters and responses aloud, they discussed and interpreted the children's dialogues and group process from the perspective of four vantage points. The authors discuss the interplay of attachment, psychodynamic, constitutional/regulatory factors, and interpersonal or group dynamics as they arise. They highlight dynamic shifts in the group process and identify defense mechanisms, both adaptive and maladaptive, as they occur. Drs. Nemiroff and DeGangi explore the emotional meanings underlying how children describe their thoughts and feelings. At times, the children had a unique perspective on problems due to their own capacity for attachment, past experiences, constitutional difficulties, and individual strengths and weaknesses. Many of the children participating in the groups had diagnoses including ADHD, Asperger's syndrome, sensory integrative dysfunction, language learning disabilities, depression, or anxiety. These developmental and emotional problems had direct impacts on each child's experience of his social world.

As Drs. DeGangi and Nemiroff discuss the clinical material with each other about the letters, they speak in plain, simple language. Their own dialogues are interspersed throughout each session's transcript. We wanted to capture the therapeutic issues and group process as they were occurring. We intentionally avoided the use of jargon in our discussions, with the exception of the formal names of primary defenses. One of the reasons we avoided theoretically laden language was because it objectifies the children whom we are talking about, rather than engaging with them in a more direct and genuine way. We try, throughout, to respect each child's individuality and avoid speaking in generalities as much as is possible. Drs. DeGangi and Nemiroff attempt to attend to the defenses used by the children while retaining focus on the emotional pain they expressed. As Winnicott (1971) has said, "the therapist should always remember to be a good host." The way in which we use our language in interacting with one another, and with the children in therapy, should reflect the humanness of the therapy experience.

The letters appearing throughout the text are written for children in these school-aged children's groups. There are some minor modifications in the letters intended for boys or for girls. At the end of each chapter, the authors suggest activities and discussion topics for use in group psychotherapy. We hope that these will prove helpful to group psychotherapists and educators who wish to use the letters in their own children's groups as a tool for participants learning about one another, developing insight, and accessing interpersonal dynamics. The suggested activities and discussion topics are intended to help children to express themselves specifically to the topic depicted in the letter. These activities include a range of approaches and media, including role-playing, drama, interview techniques, art, team-building activities, and games. They are intended to make the group experience fun and interesting while children develop skills and insight into themselves.

Drs. DeGangi and Nemiroff have worked, supervised, and taught together for many years. The collaboration of two clinicians with often differing points of view has often led to what we hope is a creative "hybridization of clinical approach." Dr. Nemiroff and Dr. DeGangi both strongly advocate "clinical pluralism." That is, different clinical orientations should enrich and not compete with one another. They hope that this spirit of collaboration and enjoyment of their differences is apparent in their dialogues. The authors believe and hope that, clinically, two-plus-two might just add up to more than four.

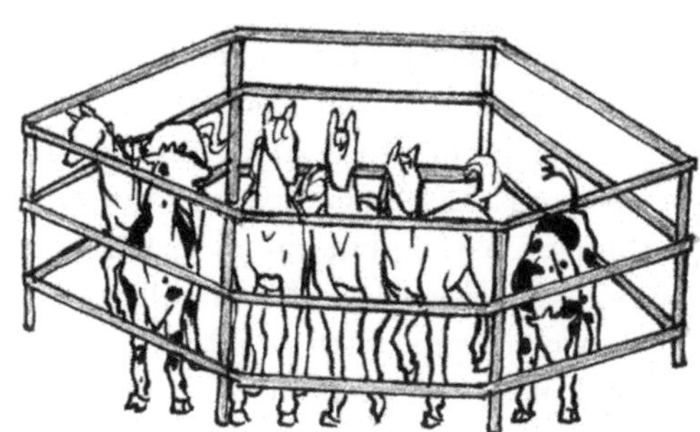

Narrative Therapy as a Treatment Modality

Narrative therapy is a powerful and effective modality in the treatment of children in psychotherapy. It has been used to address a range of childhood problems including depression, trauma, school failure, peer exclusion, and adjustment to distressing and potentially traumatic life events such as parental divorce (Freeman, Epston, & Lobovits, 1997; Smith & Nylund, 1997; Vetere & Dowling, 2005; White & Morgan, 2006). As a child engages in the therapeutic process, he brings his concerns and worries to the therapist, creating a story line that may be talked about or played out. As the child expresses himself, the narrative provides a structured window for the therapist to understand the child's inner emotional world. The therapist listens and observes in order to make sense of the meanings of the child's story, paying close attention to both verbal and non-verbal messages while seeking to go beyond surface content to understand relevant meanings for the child. As the therapist and child engage in dynamic dialogue, the child's internal world becomes more clearly defined, allowing the youngster to bring unconscious thoughts and feelings into consciousness. It also helps the child to understand that he is not *defined as* the problem, but that he is a human being who *has* a problem. Thus, this process between the therapist and child unfolds to help the child to understand himself in new and fuller ways. The emotional pace and timing of the dialogue creates a mutually shared emotional experience between therapist and child that, in itself, promotes attachment, insight, problem-solving, and mood regulation. This sharing of a mutual reality combined with being understood, mirrored, and validated by another is central to the healing process (Winnicott, 1971).

When narrative therapy is applied in a group setting, the therapist attempts to create a shared reality for the group members. In order to select topics that are relevant to group participants, Dr. DeGangi employed methods derived from qualitative and evidence-based research. Over the course of two years, she generated lists of topics that children talked about in group psychotherapy and identified recurring themes. Taking narrative therapy a step further, Dr. DeGangi introduced another "person" into the room—the letter-writer who sought advice about one of these topics. The letter-writer was created so that he would feel "real," and that the children could talk to him. The self-disclosure of this phantom child created an atmosphere that fostered the children's talking about uncomfortable things in comfortable ways. In essence, the child in the letter became a special guest who brought something that deeply troubled him to the group. His problem became, and mirrored, the group's problem. The children in the group were enabled to go through the process of self-discovery through the eyes of this phantom guest.

This method of using therapeutic letters as a narrative therapy technique has been used to help children take in and process problems and concerns (Freeman et al., 1997). Writing issues down into a letter format captures the child-language of the letter-writer into a permanent form. This is particularly helpful to the child who might be experiencing learning problems or processing deficits that make it more difficult to make sense of spoken conversational exchanges. Another, not-physically-present child, taking pen to paper asking for help, brings a safe urgency into the therapy room. The wish of another person to be helped can have a transforming effect on the listener. Wachtel eloquently depicted these kinds of statements as "emotional life-preservers in stormy seas" (Wachtel, 2001, p. 371). The result is that the child who is on the receiving end of the letter becomes valued by the letter-writer as a source of help. The listener is viewed as competent. The letter-writer beckons the listener to generate solutions to help him with what is emotionally troubling to him.

Letter-writing as a technique provides a model for talking about problems in safe ways for children in therapeutic groups. As the children listen, they see how a child gives voice to what is otherwise unsayable, without the risk of experiencing enormous shame or exposure. The words of the letter-writer are presented in an authentic and human way, so that the listener can realize that it is safe to talk about his own life too. Additionally, the listeners (group members) can see the respect the group as a whole has for the letter-writer's dilemma. The child with the problem owns his problem but is not defined solely by that problem. The wish for change in the letter-writer offers hope to the listener.

As the narrative therapy process unfolds in a group dynamic, multiple responses can occur to what might begin as a similar experience in different groups. As the children listen to the letter-writer's story, they start to respond uniquely as individuals and as members of a specific group with its own "personality." Variations in responses depend upon the child's age, gender, developmental capacities, and identification with the issue under discussion. The therapist must be vigilant to each group's personal response to the letter-writer's problem and create safety in talking about the problem. This helps children meet the challenges of listening, responding, and integrating the letter's true meanings into their own personal experiences.

As therapists, we hope that the letters in this book have an immediate impact on the children who participated in the groups. However, sometimes the anticipated positive effects take time. We also hope that future children who listen to these letters, either in group or in individual therapy, might be helped. Dr. DeGangi continued to work with a number of group members for several years after the groups ended. Some children spontaneously offered insights about the process.

Here is what one of them said on his last day of individual therapy. Rob was a participant in Boys' Group #1.

Rob: Do you know what was most memorable to me of all the things that I did here with you?

GD: Tell me, Rob. I'd love to hear what you think.

Rob: Remember those letters? I still think about those kids and wonder if their lives are better. Sometimes our advice was really bogus, but it really got under my skin. It helped me to talk about myself and realize that I wasn't alone with my problems. If it weren't for them, I probably wouldn't be telling anybody what really bugs me. I used to keep to myself and nobody knew how depressed I was all the time, but the kids in my group knew about it and so do you.

GD: I'm so glad that you're telling me this, Rob. It helps me to know what worked for you. You have really grown as a person from coming here and I'm so glad that I could be a part of your life. Stay in touch with me, Rob.

Rob: I will. I'm thinking of calling William from the group to get together. He was a good egg.

References

Freeman, J., Epston, D., & Lobovits, D. (1997). *Playful approaches to serious problems*. New York: W.W. Norton & Co.

Smith, C., & Nylund, D. (Eds.). (1997). *Narrative therapies with children and adolescents*. New York: Guilford Press.

Vetere, A., & Dowling, E. (Eds.). (2005). *Narrative therapies with children and their families*. New York: Routledge.

Wachtel, E. F. (2001). The language of becoming: Helping children change how they think about themselves. *Family Process*, *40*(4), 369–384.

White, M., & Morgan, A. (2006). *Narrative therapy with children and their families*. Adelaide, South Australia: Dulwich Centre Publications.

Winnicott, D. W. (1971). *Playing and reality*. Harmondsworth: Penguin.

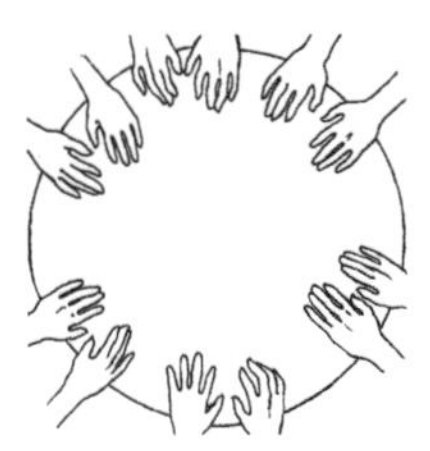

Cast of Characters

Boys' Group #1

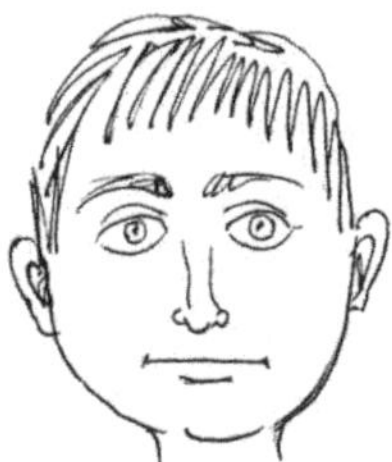

Henry was a lonely, anxious, and shy 10-year-old boy. He had no friends and spent long hours isolated in his bedroom, either reading fantasy novels or playing computer games. He was quite intelligent, yet had trouble making conversation with other people. Although not diagnosed as such, he presented as a child with Asperger's syndrome. He was awkward socially and had a distant interpersonal quality. He frequently gazed away when talking with others and his affect was flat. He was a very sweet youngster who evoked in others the desire to connect with him emotionally.

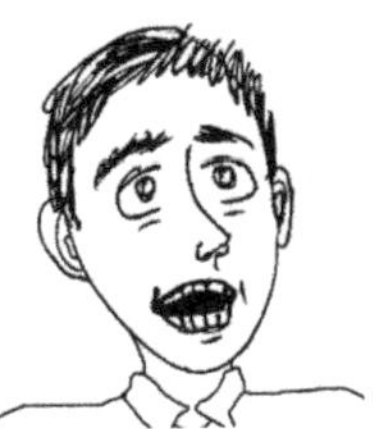

Jacob, 10 years old, identified strongly with his Orthodox Jewish background. It was rare to have a conversation without him bringing up something about his Jewish religion and identity. He was bright and was well informed about many different topics. He had an off-kilter sense of humor and liked playing practical jokes on others. His jokes would often take a wrong turn and annoy his peers. As a result he had few friends and, sadly, his parents found him obnoxious, oppositional, and very difficult to be around. Although Jacob seemed to be laughing most of the time, there was an anxious and very troubled child who lived underneath the surface.

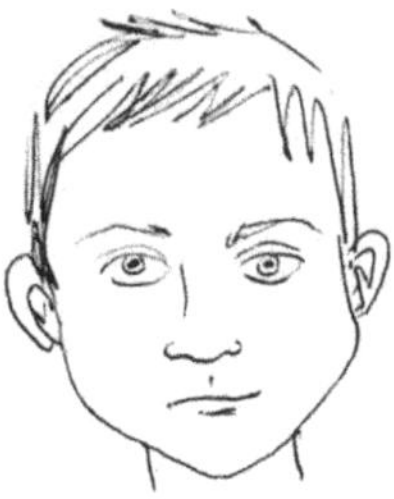

Javier was an 11-year-old boy who could have been a "poster child" for Asperger's syndrome. When he first began the group, he was so hypersensitive to the sounds of other children talking and having fun that he would flee from the room, cover his ears, and complain: "It's too loud in here!" Javier was brilliant and loved reading. He almost always had his head buried in a book in the waiting room and the therapist often needed to tell him to put it away during group sessions. When Javier participated in the group conversation, he tended to soliloquize. Javier was content to be isolated. He showed no desire for friends when he first began the group. Over time, he came to view the other boys in the group as his best friends.

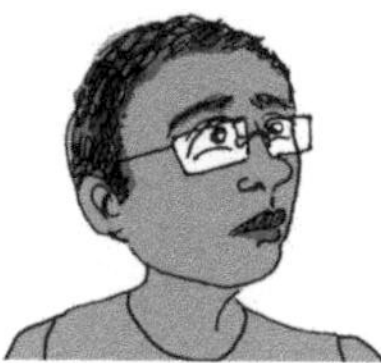

Duncan, an 11-year-old boy on the Autistic Spectrum, needed much encouragement to join in the group conversation. Frequently self-absorbed, he would pick on himself with his fingers and pull on his ears. During group, he would sit off in a corner alone. When he did participate, it was usually about an idiosyncratic topic, or his obsession with "Captain Underpants." When he engaged in the group conversation, he easily went off on tangents.

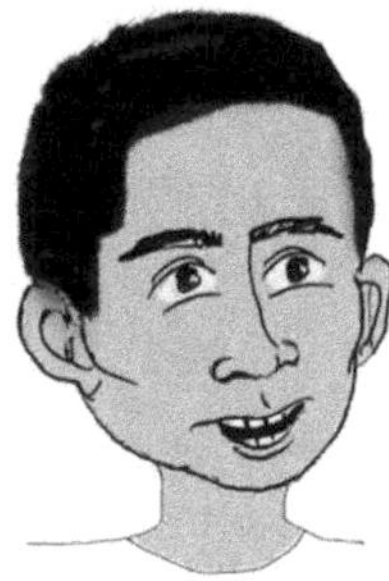

Tyrone was an 11-year-old boy who had multiple motor and language problems as a result of a brain tumor that had been removed as a young boy. He was an odd-looking child with a small frame and awkward body movements. When he was anxious, he would dart his eyes about and cower. Tyrone found it very difficult to talk about anything, especially his thoughts or feelings, regardless of the topic.

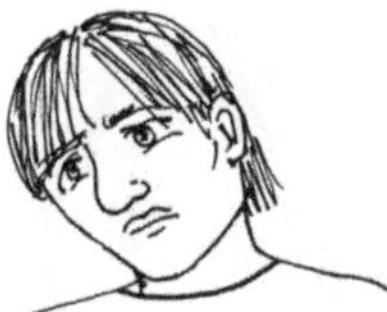

Aaron was an arrogant, bossy, 11-year-old boy with attention-deficit hyperactivity disorder (ADHD). He had to be in charge and constantly jockeyed for the spotlight. He was frequently loud, obnoxious, and domineering, constantly in motion, tipping his chair back, pacing the room, and grabbing things. Despite his bossy and bullying demeanor, he was an emotionally needy child who hungered for the group leader's attention and relentlessly asked for snacks. He was an exemplar of the kind of youngster who could not take "no" for an answer.

Boys' Group #2

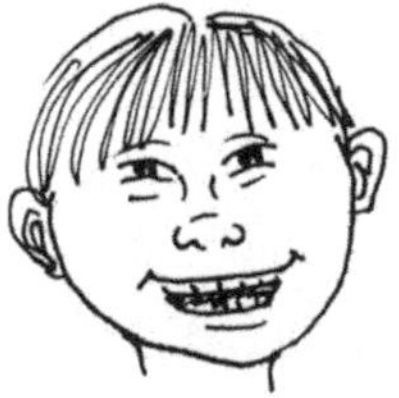

Aidan, a nine-year-old boy, looked more like a seven-and-a-half-year-old. He was scrawny and short for his age. He had severe attention-deficit disorder (ADD) with hyperactivity and impulsivity. He needed 100% supervision from his parents, or else he could get into hot water within moments. He could be outlandish and outrageous in aggressive and oppositional ways. He was a very frightened child behind these behaviors, who experienced an unremitting level of internal distress and such frustration that he was angry with himself for not being able to control his own impulses. He saw the problem, he knew the problem, and he hated himself for having the problem. Although his parents found Aidan to be a hard-to-love child, he had a sweet and sensitive side to him. In calm moments, he could be empathic and loving, but usually he quickly switched to the impulsive, out-of-control child that he usually was.

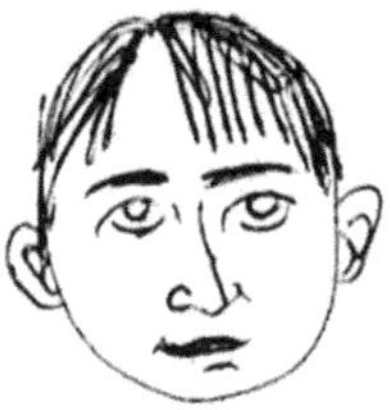

Julian, a notably somber 10-year-old boy, desperately wanted friends but quickly alienated them. He frequently found himself in difficult situations in which other boys would become aggressive toward him, pick on him physically, and tease him mercilessly. Sadly, this happened in almost every social situation. Julian was also hypersensitive on both sensory and emotional levels, and so would quickly dissolve into tears. His sensitivity only worsened his social plight.

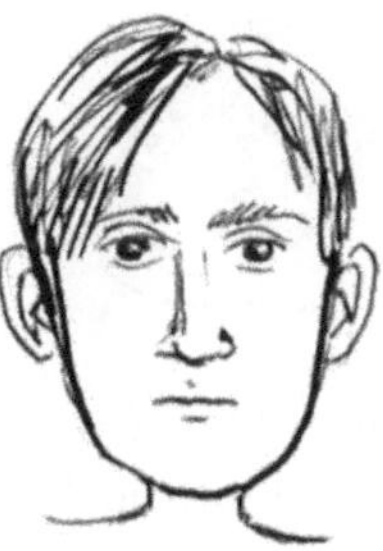

Kevin was a 10-year-old boy with Asperger's syndrome. He, too, was quite bright but had no social sense: he simply could not read the social cues of others. Kevin had many talents, including acting and music, but in the sports arena he was uncoordinated and would struggle. At school, he was often picked on because he seemed "un-cool" to the other boys. His difficulties reading social cues often put him in situations in which he was taunted, bullied, or provoked. He had no idea how to get himself out of these situations in skillful ways, and usually did things to make it worse. He was a sad victim of his own ineptitude.

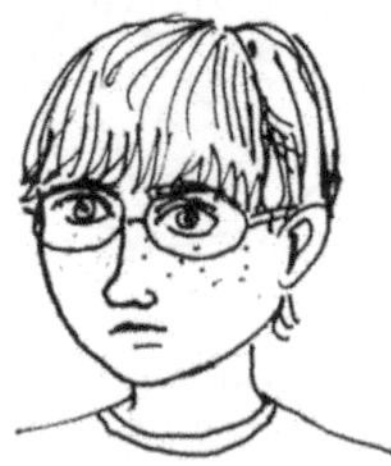

Ian, by age 10, had struggled for years to try and fit in with his peers, always without success. Already, at such a young age, he identified with Goth* dress and tried to look tough. Underneath this exterior demeanor was an emotionally fragile young boy. Ian had ADHD and difficulty following conversations. He was learning that if he dominated any conversation, he would not have to worry about listening to others and responding to what they had said. Ian had a tendency to fall apart easily, to have tantrums at home, and to become aggressive when overwhelmed.

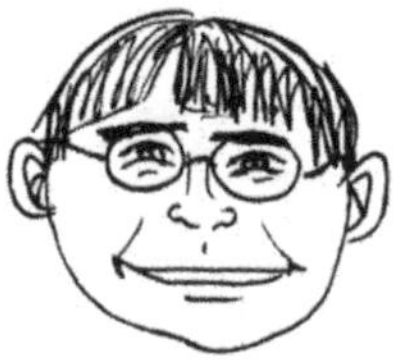

Manuel was an 11-year-old boy who struggled mightily to fit in with others, but who frequently failed for several reasons. His ADD often got him into trouble, without his

---

* "Goth" refers to a social subgroup of youngsters who identify with their social, and perceived emotional, differentness by flaunting their status as misfits. Goths transform their pain into an attention-getting "in your face" attitude shown in their usually all-black dress, outlandish hairstyles, and overall demeanor. They wear their depression as a badge. It is palpable, visible, and untouchable.

understanding how he got into the situation; for example, he might take a manicure set to school in his wallet and then find himself suspended for his unacceptable behavior and poor judgment. Many times he got entangled in bad social situations that often were partly of his own making. He would then make matters worse by defending himself over and over again, until the school principal needed to be called in to sort things out. Manuel was overweight and physically inactive; this often made him the target of teasing. He was extremely verbal, had a strong interest in science fiction, and seemed to get along best with adults. Mid-year he had a scheduling conflict and moved to Boys' Group #1.

Boys' Group #3

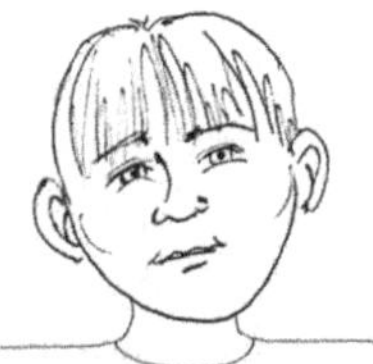

Justin was a lovably, eccentric 11-year-old boy who had something to say about almost everything. He had an unusual perspective on the world and often confused the nuances of social situations. He was hypersensitive to touch and sound, enough so to run from the group room whenever he felt overwhelmed. He would easily become overwrought when over-stimulated both emotionally or by sensory stimulation.

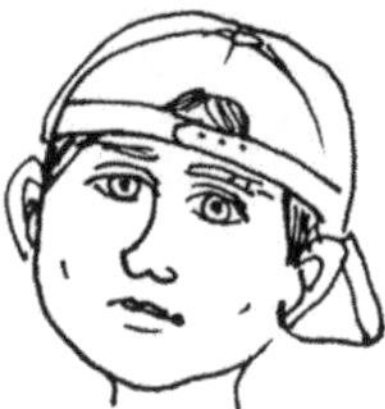

Nate, a 10-year-old boy as sweet as he might be, could nevertheless become very impulsive and do outlandish things without thinking. He would get himself into trouble and never quite know how it could have happened. Afterwards he would always feel remorseful and could then problem-solve what he might do the next time. However, the results of this problem-solving always failed him when the next difficult situation would arise. Nate was thus always on intimate terms with remorse, regret, and a sense of failure: "I messed up AGAIN!"

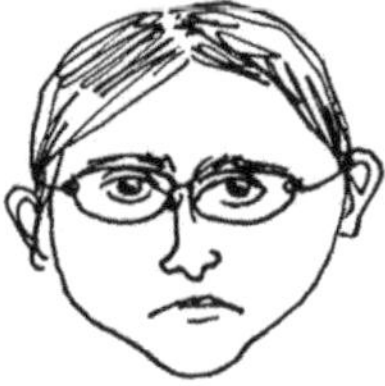

Oliver was a brilliant but vulnerable 10-year-old boy who easily surpassed his peers in all subjects. His poignant depression was palpable. He believed, at his sad core, that he did not fit in with anybody. He wore his hair particularly long and had wire-rimmed glasses that also distinguished him from his peers. Symbolic of his alienated self-perception, he had developed a close identification with Godzilla. When he talked about Godzilla, he became hyper-excited. As the year progressed, Oliver expressed deep feelings of depression, and sometimes suicidal thoughts. Godzilla was undeniably powerful and noticeable, but he was also a creature from whom everyone wanted to get away.

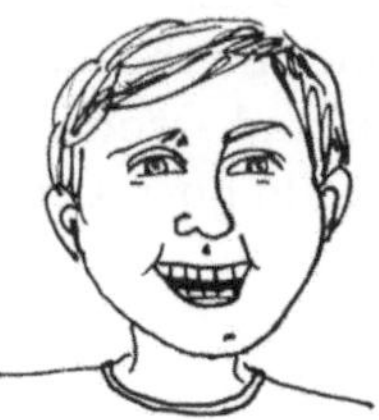

Jamie was an odd 10-year-old boy with a diagnosis of pervasive developmental disorder (PDD). He was uncoordinated and constantly spilled things on himself and others. He had numerous allergies, especially food allergies that required special attention. Jamie was a markedly messy eater and always seemed to be smeared with catsup on his face and shirt. He would get so excited talking about certain topics that he could not shift his attention away to the task or conversation at hand. Despite all his difficulties, Jamie had a sense of humor that served him well and helped him be an appealing child.

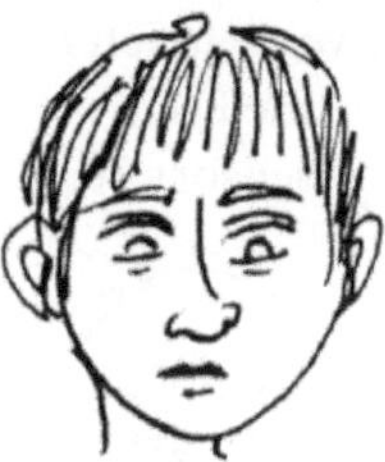

Corey was a cute 10-year-old boy with ADHD. He always came a few minutes late to group and would enter with gusto, knocking over chairs and creating a general ruckus. He was in constant motion, tipping his chair back, moving and touching things, and wiggling around. Corey was exceptionally distractible; he noticed every sound in the environment and consequently could not distinguish important from unimportant sounds. Everything was equal. Sometimes Corey would be in his own world, as if in a fog, and would need to be reoriented to what his group was talking about or doing. Corey often got the giggles and would be overly silly at times. The other boys found this both annoying and over-stimulating.

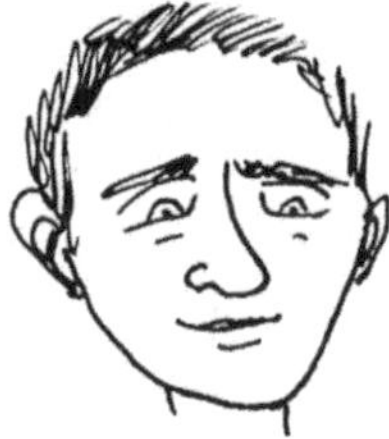

Leo was 10 years old and had Asperger's syndrome. The boys in the group tended not to like him, and they often did things to socially sabotage him when he did do something nice or was kind to others. He was frequently a braggart and know-it-all, which was off-putting. He became quickly over-stimulated in the group. This usually escalated to aggression or physical disruption. Often the therapist needed to help him pull himself together by taking him out of the group room and helping him organize his behavior. When alone with the therapist, he became very sweet and receptive to feedback. Over time, Leo made a great deal of progress in learning to control his impulsivity, aggression, and the need to be the center of attention.

Girls' Group #1

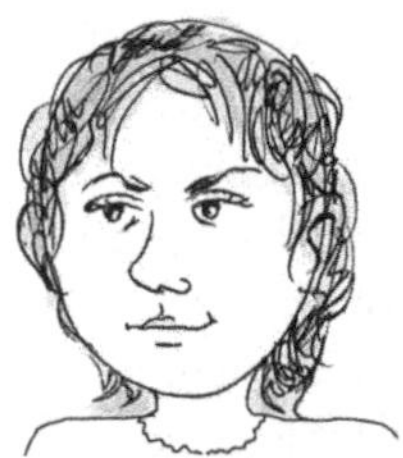

Mallory was 12 years old and had a severe non-verbal learning disability. She was completely stumped by social interactions and often would not comprehend even the most basic relational dynamics. The only thing she seemed to understand was slapstick humor. After two years in the group, she still did not know the names of the other girls. She would sit hunched over, anxiously twirling her hair, speaking only when directly asked a question. On the surface, she appeared to be a very sweet, overwhelmed child. However, she had a very dark side filled with sinister thoughts about death and killing people. Mallory had a collection of china dolls that she often brought to group to share. These were a metaphor for her intensely fragile self-identity. It poignantly seemed her only way (without using words) to help her group-mates understand how she felt about herself.

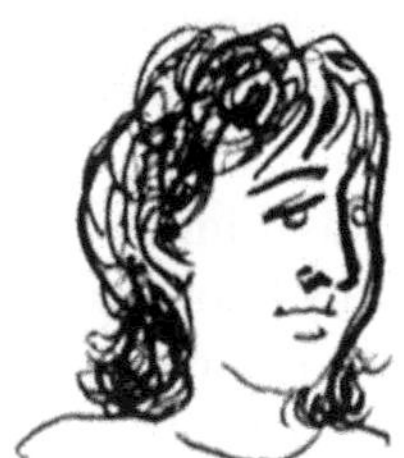

Rosa was a 12-year-old girl who was also diagnosed with Asperger's syndrome. She was a highly concrete thinker who relied on extreme structure as her only way to field social interactions. She processed social interactions in a highly rigid manner. It was nearly impossible for her to consider another person's perspective. She interacted with others by being highly scripted and stilted. Without a rigid, predictable, structure, she quickly became overwhelmed. Rosa was an only child and was used to getting her way. Her self-centered nature frequently and unsurprisingly interfered with her ability to make and sustain friendships. When she did become playful and more spontaneous, she repeated the same joke over and over until all humor was lost. Her idea of a good "joke" was wanting to pour water over somebody's head in the group.

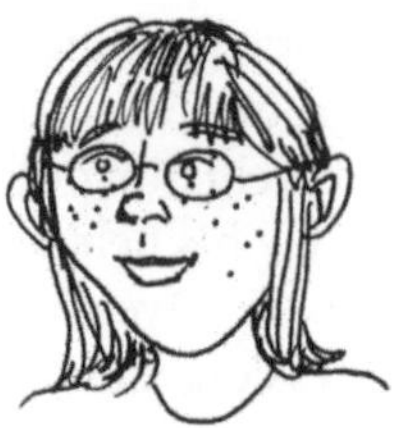

Crystal, a very troubled 12-year-old girl, was adopted from Romania when she was four years old. She had fetal alcohol syndrome and severe ADHD with impulsivity. She was an engaging and compelling child who could tell a good story about home or school life. Crystal was quite aware of the trouble that she got into on a daily basis and frequently came to group asking what she should do to solve these problems. During calm moments, she was able to articulate and think through what might be a good solution to a problem situation. More typically, Crystal escalated quickly into an overdrive state. In her more primitive interactive moments, she might repeatedly roar like a lion in someone's face. At home, she would clog the toilet with rolls of toilet paper or bite on a table edge surface like a dog. Her parents found her exhausting to manage. She was an only child and had no friends. Other parents often did not want their youngsters to play with Crystal. She was endlessly at the mercy of herself.

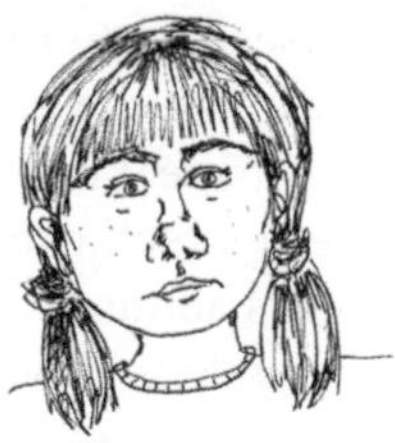

Amy was a 12-year-old girl with multiple physical and cognitive challenges. She had had many surgeries over her life, including facial reconstruction for a cleft palate. Amy was sensitive about her appearance and sometimes devastated when boys at school made fun of her looks. She often bumped into things or fell down on purpose to get attention, and then called out "Ow! I hurt myself!" to the group. She was using this strategy to express her inner pain behaviorally. Amy had a great deal of difficulty knowing what to talk about in group and usually focused on concrete topics such as going to a restaurant or her latest basketball game. Amy's primary relationship in the group was with the therapist, to whom she was quite attached.

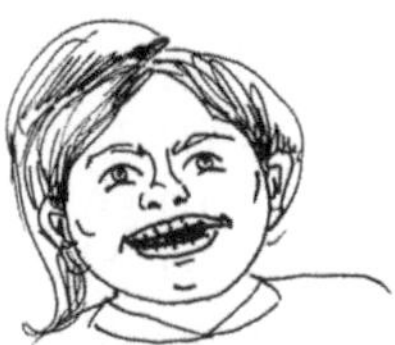

Abby was an over-anxious 12-year-old girl with significant language learning disabilities. She frequently expressed her emotional distress about being overlooked and not listened to by others. She lacked the social and language skills to navigate even the simplest of social interactions. Abby was at a chronic loss as to how to break into groups or know what to say, and needed considerable prompting to help her form her thoughts to share with others. When she did speak, she did not elaborate her ideas.

Girls' Group #2

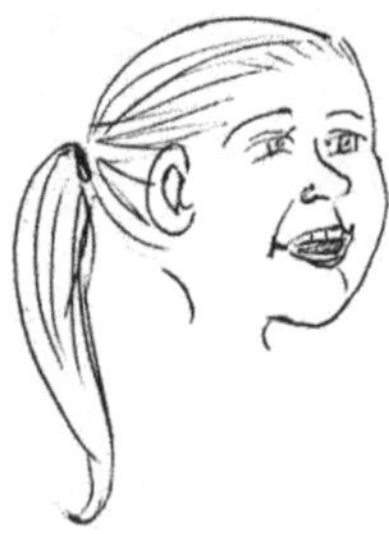

Chelsea, an adopted nine-year-old girl with ADD, often seemed to be on a different wavelength than the other girls in the group. She frequently seemed disengaged and looked about the room for visual stimulation. Although she could talk intelligently about the problems of others, she brought very little of herself to the group. She had an empty, ghost-like quality. Despite her musical and athletic talents, she seemed to be a youngster with little substance to her, as if she could not internalize the reality of her own being. She had an older sister who was multiply-handicapped and who could neither speak nor walk. Her home life centered on the older sister's needs and Chelsea was frequently overlooked. This may well have contributed to her spectral presence.

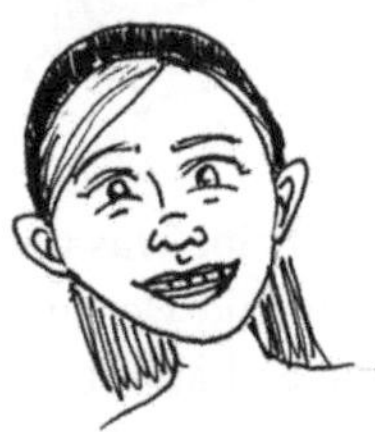

Maya was a sweet and lonely nine-year-old girl. Her parents had just moved the family to the area, and Maya was devastated at losing her old friends. She was having a hard time entering a new group of children at school. She had become shy and withdrawn, even though she had been quite personable before the move. Despite her many talents, Maya disliked herself and was sure that no one else liked her either. She was difficult to draw out of her sadness; she had locked up her vitality.

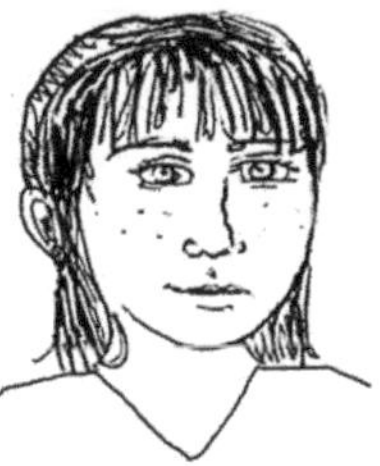

Ellen was a shy, nine-year-old stutterer. She was also very awkward physically and seemed to disappear into the background unless invited to participate. She had a great deal of performance anxiety and low self-esteem. Ellen's "stay-in-the-background," wallflower adaptation only served to reinforce her isolation and her sense of herself as negligible.

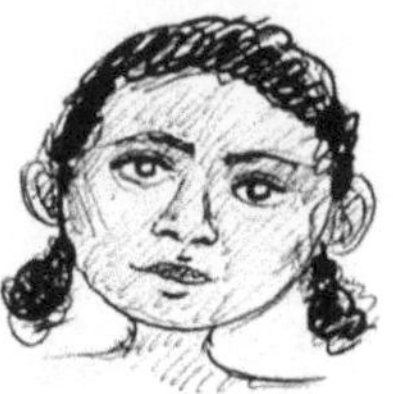

Latisha was a very beautiful girl with dark flowing hair, dark eyes, and lovely brown skin. Sadly, by age nine, she often talked about hating her looks, wanting to be blond and blue-eyed like Briana, another girl in the group. She was fearful of, and anxious about, all kinds of things: elevators, a bad man following her, or someone breaking into her house. She did not have the ability to like herself, accept herself, and appreciate herself for who she was.

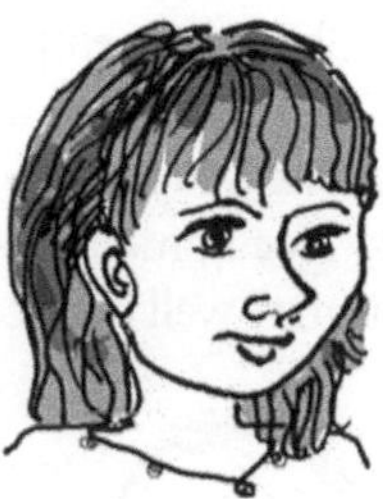

Briana was an adopted nine-year-old girl. She was perky, showy, and narcissistic. She often flaunted her pretty looks to others and would wear pinks and baby-blues to accentuate her blond hair and blue eyes. She often bragged about her most recent acquisition or achievement and was prone to exclude others intentionally. Already, at age nine, she had a "Queen Bee Wannabee" attitude. She always had something to say about others' behavior but hated any attention on her own faux-pas. She managed her secret sense of being deeply flawed by focusing on the flaws of others.

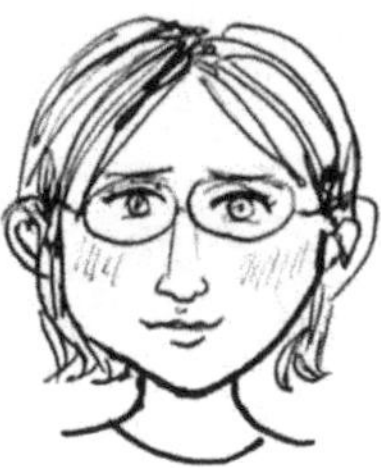

Danielle was nine years old and tiny, with heart problems that truly worried her. She had Asperger's syndrome as well and was intensely preoccupied with figurines that she had collected. She often came into group with her face buried in a comic book and would need many prompts to get her to put it away. When she spoke, it was always a long soliloquy that pushed the other girls away. Even when they said things like, "Get to the point" or "Can you finish it up already?" she would jabber on. Closeness in relationships was clearly very hard for her and kept her an isolated misfit.

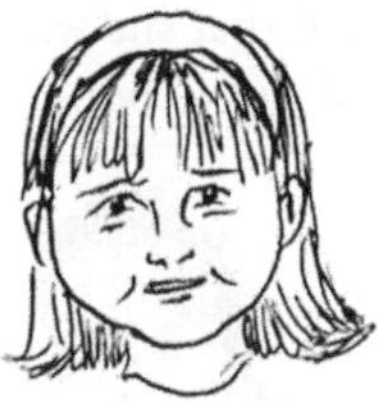

Annie was a very shy, withdrawn nine-year-old girl who suffered from severe seasonal affective disorder. During the winter months, she frequently wrote very creative but dark poetry and depressing stories. Despite her withdrawn nature, she was also quite restless and might sit in group expressing a high degree of restlessness and agitation, rocking her chair too and fro when emotionally charged material was being discussed.

Girls' Group #3

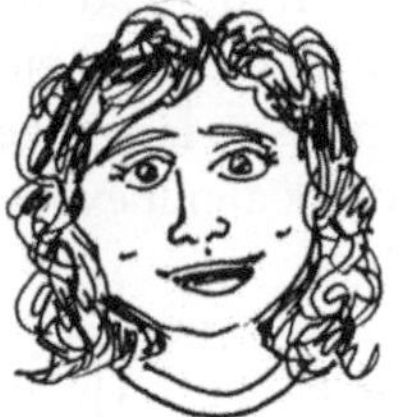

Ashley was an appealing 11-year-old girl with the slight and agile physique of a gymnast. Her diminutive stature notwithstanding, Ashley was often in the middle of conflicts with peers or wherever the action was and, certainly was not overlooked. She became quickly agitated and anxious even as she craved intensity in interactions. She would often wring her hands during group sessions or kick her legs as she listened to others. Despite her interest in others' problems, Ashley found it very difficult to talk about herself and would quickly change the subject, diverting it from her. She came from a home with very supportive parents, but who were themselves highly anxious and disorganized.

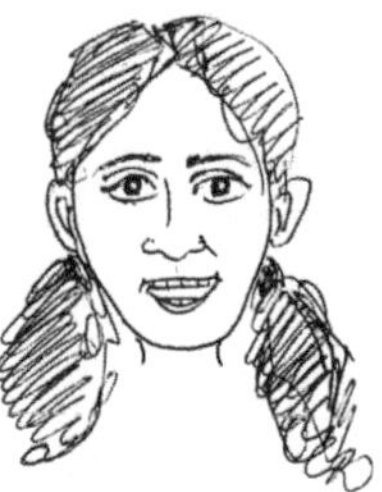

Deborah was an 11-year-old girl with Asperger's syndrome. She looked haunted and seemed to live in a fantasy world. Her avid, almost compulsive, reading fueled her fantasy life. However, she also had moments when she would indeed hear voices that told her to do obsessive things. Deborah was frequently self-absorbed, lost in her own thoughts that were usually unrelated to the group's agenda. Conversations with Deborah tended to be one-sided, yet she rarely actually shared much about herself. She worked hard to maintain a highly private profile. Deborah often felt that she was being wronged by others and seemed preoccupied with how unfair the world was to her.

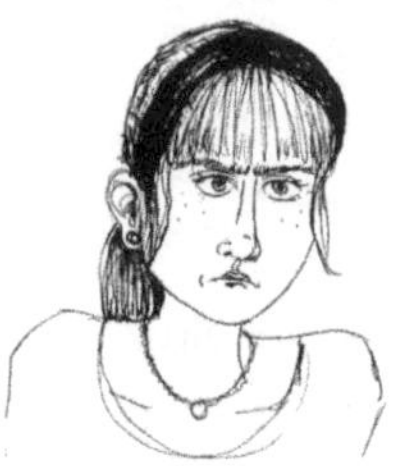

Gillian was a complex, multiply-involved, 11-year-old girl who suffered from cerebral palsy, ADD, and learning disabilities. She strongly identified herself as an athlete and sports enthusiast despite the fact that sports were very difficult for her to do. She had very few other interests and had a hard time participating in most group activities. Usually she would roam the room, disengaged from the group process, and needed a great deal of attention from the group therapist to find ways to stay involved. In addition, Gillian's speech was very difficult to understand. Even though she had a lot to say when we talked about the letters, the other girls would ignore her because her expressive language was so slow and labored. Gillian had a quick temper and would frequently talk about exploding.

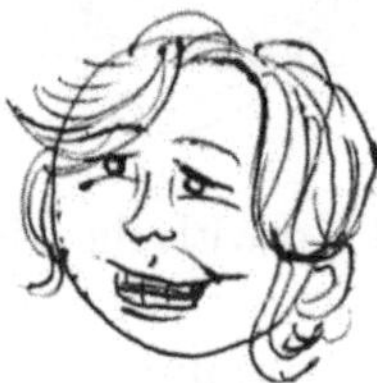

Alexis, who had severe ADHD, was an adopted 10-year-old girl from Russia. She was small for her age and looked as if she might have had fetal alcohol syndrome. Alexis was impulsive and immature and frequently grabbed things in the room that were not part of the group's activities. She could be rather disdainful of others and self-centered. She would grab things and call "dibs" to be first. Her interactions were quite young for her age and her favorite thing to do was to play with the dollies.

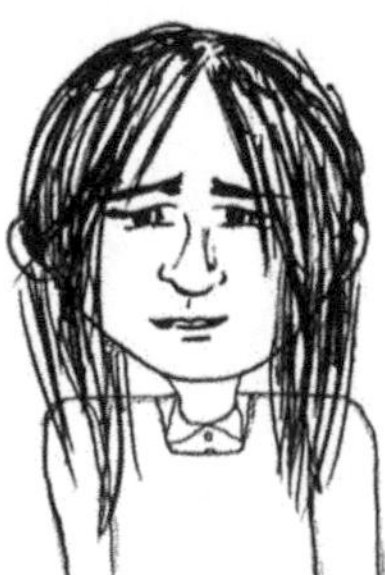

Kendra was a 10-year-old bi-racial girl (Caucasian/African American) adopted into a Caucasian family. She had gender identity problems and ADHD. She consistently came to group dressed and acting like a boy. She had no other interests other than sports. Kendra often had nothing to say about herself and seemed like an empty shell of a person. She came from a home in which there were no behavioral limits and few rules that were enforced.

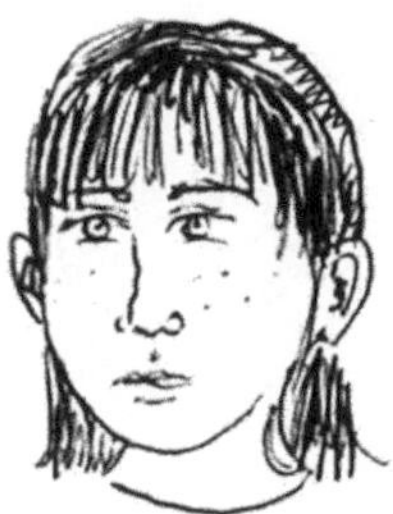

Elizabeth was 11 years old and quite immature. She had severe language and executive functioning problems that caused her to have no idea what to say to others. Her default response was "I don't know." Her lack of ability to form ideas or think through situations produced a great deal of anxiety, as if she were rather distressed at her own inability to express her feelings or ideas. Thus, she was locked inside herself, unable to express herself and become known by the other girls.

Girls' Group #4

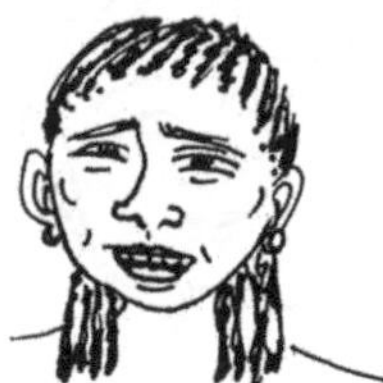

Tori was a nine-year-old girl with severe obsessive-compulsive disorder. During group sessions, she constantly pulled out pens and pencils, lay them on her lap, stashed them in her pockets, and asked repetitive questions about Sharpie™ pens. It was very difficult to set limits on this behavior. Tori was fun-loving but had no clue as to how to organize play with her peers. Her ability to relate to the other girls was severely compromised. Tori's play tended to be notably immature. When the group would discuss various topics, her typical response was concrete and rigid.

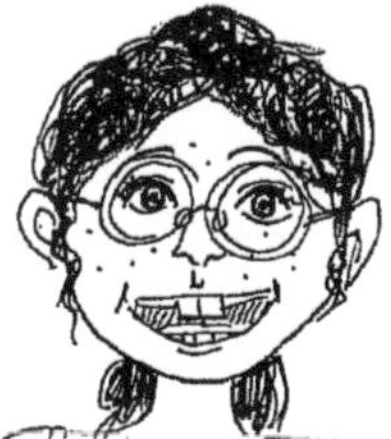

Caitlin, a tiny, wiry, odd-looking eight-year-old girl with thick glasses, was a rather talkative youngster. She could easily get started on a talking riff and could not read social cues that told her when to stop. Caitlin could become very silly and then quickly escalate to outlandish and annoying behavior. She sometimes purposely fell out of her chair, pressed her face up against others while laughing loudly, or picked her nose and rubbed it on the other children's clothes. This behavior symbolized how she considered herself repellant. During calm moments, she was capable of being insightful and friendly, but these times were rare. Caitlin had a chaotic home life: her parents were recently divorced and her mother was seriously overwhelmed and depressed.

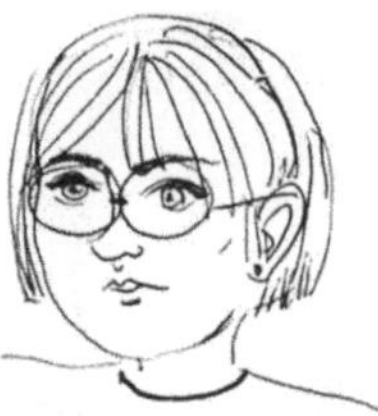

Morgan was a pretty nine-year-old girl with gleaming blue eyes. She was extremely shy and rarely talked, always struggling with the basics of what to say to peers. She appeared anxious and overwhelmed, but underneath was a festering anger. At home, she exploded whenever she felt that things were unfairly balanced in favor of her little sister. She would do devious things to get back at others, especially when she felt that she had been wronged. Usually this took the form of telling a tall tale or lying by asserting that someone had done something to her.

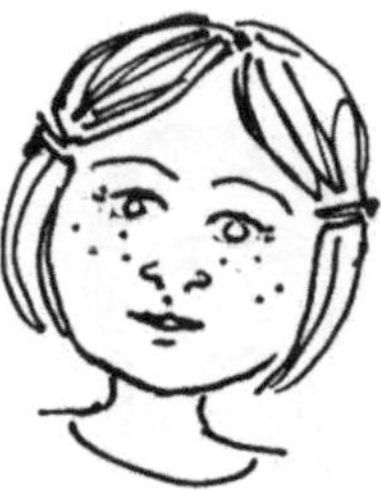

Hannah, an anxious nine-year-old girl, had a history of social phobia. She was very quiet and shy, breathing audibly in an anxious manner during the few times she spoke in her group sessions. She had hypersensitivities to sound and touch, and often pulled her chair away from the intimacy of the circle to maintain the safety of her self-imposed isolation. During the time she participated in group, she remained aloof and detached, showing little interest in the other children. She would, however, frequently sit next to the group leader and seemed attached to her.

Girls' Group #5

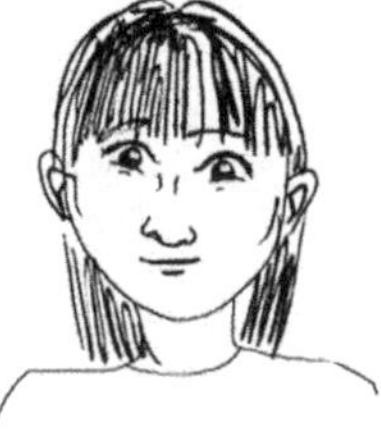

Jacqueline was a compelling 11-year-old girl with an interesting and curious mind. She struggled with ADHD, while her fraternal twin was the "golden" girl. Jacqueline loved adventure. However, she would easily get side-tracked by her own ideas and find herself in difficult situations wondering how in the world she got there. She would be impulsive and do outlandish things, but always with the intention of being kind. She might climb a high tree to save an abandoned bird, for instance, but then fall onto the ground injuring her back. Jacqueline often looked lost in thought. She loved nature and often brought interesting bugs and other little creatures into group to share, and once decorated her hair and blouse with cicada shells. Adults loved talking to Jacqueline, but children had a hard time knowing how to connect to her singularity.

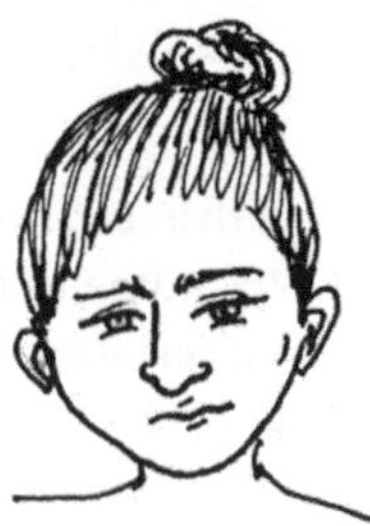

Nadia, an 11-year-girl, was adopted from Russia at age three. She was a diminutive, shy, and inhibited girl who looked chronically afraid. She was clearly anxious and needed a great deal of help to find the nerve to speak up in her group. She desperately wanted to be liked but had few skills even to get noticed by others. She usually stood on the outskirts of group and needed support and guidance in order to join in; she did not know how to do it. As she entered fifth grade, she began to get into trouble in school, accepting "double-dares" to win the grace of popular girls. She was desperate to be accepted because she felt so very different. Nadia was a daydreamer and often forgot the things that she wanted to say. She also had difficulty following the conversational line. With considerable help, she could come to express her ideas and feelings.

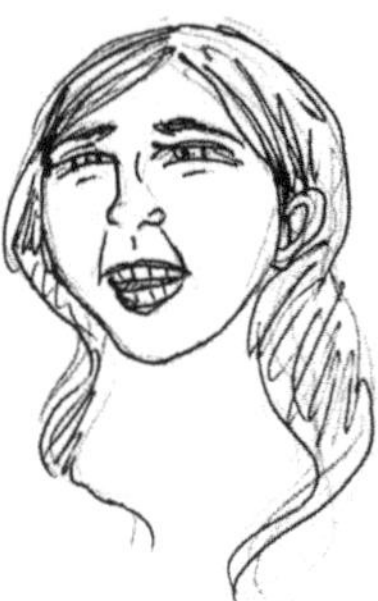

Brooke was an attractive 10-year-old girl with green eyes and ashen blond hair. She was adopted and was an only child. She had tremendous difficulty managing her ADHD and was frequently bossy, impulsive, and controlling. She had quite a hard time finishing activities and quickly got angry if she felt rushed. If given a leader role, she would thrive, but she could not tolerate sharing any control with others. Most of the girls in the group viewed Brooke cautiously and felt that she was self-centered, in part because she almost always needed to bring the discussion back to herself. Brooke often boasted about her skills at horseback riding. Brooke had a narcissistic quality that made it difficult for the other girls to like her. She seemed to have little or no capacity to care about the other girls' perspectives and was often incapable of empathy. Despite this, over the years she was in group therapy, she eventually became responsive to treatment, demonstrated the capacity for warmth, and developed a close attachment to the group therapist.

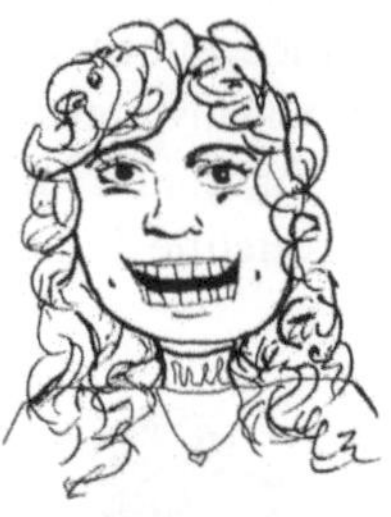

Brittany was an 11-year-old adopted girl with a terrible history of abuse during the first four years of life. She was moved from one foster home to the next. At last very loving and supportive parents adopted her. Brittany was a serious collector of trinkets, dolls, and "stuff." These were the things that she was most apt to share, finding it difficult to share her authentic feelings about herself. Brittany often talked about all kinds of things in a few minutes' time, skittering from topic to topic: boys whom she liked, going to the movies, her latest acquisition, and so on. Her conversation was empty and often like a word-salad. Frequently Brittany got into the thick of social conflicts, seriously missed the nuances of the situation, and then responded by becoming highly emotional herself. Brittany was preoccupied with hatred of her birth-mother and often became angry quickly, without knowing why.

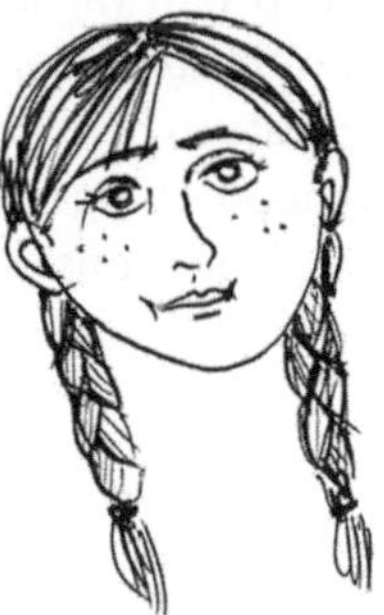

Melissa, a worried and anxious nine-year-old girl, felt all alone and struggled with notable mood instability. She often fell apart for no apparent reason and would scream at her parents over small "offenses." She did not want to be part of the group when it began, but quickly saw it as a place where she could be accepted for who she was. Soon she began sharing intimate details of her personal life with the group and used it well as a source of support.

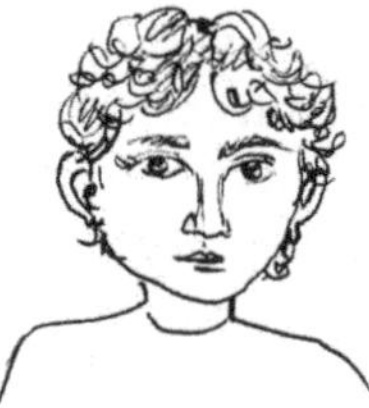

Greer, a nine-year-old girl, was beginning to show signs of a mood disorder, fluctuating between sad, depressed moments and angry, explosive behavior. Most of the time she was very quiet and rarely said anything in group unless facilitated by the therapist. Her mother was blind and struggled mightily with the isolation of this experience. Greer joined her group mid-year.

Acknowledgments

Many people have helped us in writing this book. First and foremost, we would like to thank the many children and families with whom we have worked over the years. They have been our best teachers in discovering the most effective ways to help children who experience emotional challenges. Without them, this book would not have been possible.

We have had the good fortune of working in a variety of settings that have allowed us to grow as professionals. Dr. DeGangi would like to thank all of her colleagues at ITS (Integrated Therapy Services): PALSS (Psychological and Learning Support Services), Inc. in Kensington, MD. These colleagues have provided ongoing support and insight that have allowed her to blend different therapeutic perspectives including cognitive–behavioral therapy and mind–body approaches with psychodynamic therapies in the practice of group psychotherapy for children. She would like to thank Dr. Bruce Pickle, Dr. Griff Doyle, Dr. Daniel Griffin, and Ms. Lenni Snyder, who were her coleaders in group psychotherapy. Their insights and skills helped her to grow as a therapist and to develop the ideas that created the therapeutic technique for this book.

Dr. Nemiroff would like to thank Dr. Jane Annunziata, Dr. Douglas Romberg, and Mariby Johns, LCSW, his ever-supportive colleagues. Thanks also to the many other colleagues who have shown me the way toward plurality in psychotherapy, toward the integration of approaches and orientations necessary to truly help our patients. I have learned, through many wise colleagues, that all human beings are unified wholes and not compartmentalized creatures. We are only complete when viewed through many lenses simultaneously. A special thanks to Vivian Boul, LCSW, who set me on the path.

Always above all, I want to thank my loving wife, Lin, for her boundless support for this and for all my endeavors. Thank you for unselfishly putting up with all those endless hours of writing, editing, and that always-present sore back from being hunched over the computer! And, always and forever, thank you for our beautiful partnership.

We give many thanks to Ziza Craig, Rachel Jordan, and Sara Squires for the beautifully drawn illustrations in this book. We also thank Lisa Lewis who contributed the very insightful and creative cartoons that appear throughout the book.

The dialogues that appear in this book are actual conversations recorded and transcribed for the purposes of this text. The names and pertinent identifying information of children and their families have been disguised to protect their identities.

Last but not least, Dr. DeGangi wishes to thank her loving husband, Robert Dickey, who endured many hours of listening to her as she formulated ideas for this book. She is very grateful for his unconditional support and encouragement for her professional endeavors.

PART I
Identity Formation and Understanding Oneself

Who am I?

The central question of any human being is: "Who am I?" The child develops an internal picture of himself as he learns and defines "who I am." The perception of oneself develops in conjunction with an understanding of "who I am" in relation to other people. It is a lifelong task that begins in childhood and continues throughout life as one changes. The question of "who I am" changes and evolves throughout the life span.

This first collection of letters gives us the opportunity to see through a window into the child's mind of how children form a sense of self. By viewing children's responses to letters about identity, we can witness and hopefully facilitate the group members' work to understand this primary question. Therefore, the letters in Part I focus on the development of identity in latency and pre-adolescent-aged children. The letters are intended to evoke issues common to children with social problems, particularly their feelings of competence and vulnerability, as well as how they learn to cope with understanding what it means to have ADHD or other learning or social problems.

Many children with identity problems lack the social competence to navigate the peer dynamics that occur on the playground, at school, and other social gatherings. As a result, they rarely get positive feedback from peers to help form a stronger and more secure sense of self. They may also lack the language and conceptual understanding to think about their internal self and their identity, even as they are in the midst of this age-normative struggle. Without adequate mirroring from peers or an observing ego from within, the sense of self can be easily compromised (Gemelli, 1996; Leiberg & Anders, 2006).

The Dear Kids' Club letters in Part I focus on helping children understand more about their learning styles and personalities. While their identities include their particular social and learning problems, their difficulties do not *define* who they are. In other words, a child needs to learn that she *isn't* her attention-deficit disorder, but that her attention-deficit disorder has an impact on her, and therefore requires understanding as to how it *contributes* to her self-identity. The group therapists, through the letters in Part I, worked with the children to try to emphasize the development of insight, with particular focus on the past, current, and evolving sense of self. Many children who participate in group psychotherapy often experience difficulties with attentional focus, anxiety, mood regulation, transitions, and organizational skills. Some children also have sensory integrative problems that impact relationships with others. For example, a child may have tactile sensitivities and cannot tolerate the proximity of peers, or the child is easily over-stimulated by group activity. The letters in Part I were designed to help them to understand what their needs are and to generate strategies to help themselves. This approach was intended to help free these children from being prisoners of their disabilities and to become better able to understand "Who am I?"

Dr. DeGangi and Dr. Nemiroff discuss in dialogue with each other the interaction of these constitutional/regulatory factors, their impact on individual psychodynamics, and conversely, the impact of individual psychodynamics on the child's management of constitutional/regulatory problems. In addition, the interplay of the above factors with group process is part of their discussions. The dialogue approach and this integrated philosophy inform all the clinical dialogue of the book. Just as group therapy consists of ongoing dialogues, Drs. Nemiroff and DeGangi engage in ongoing dialogue throughout each group therapy session as they review each transcript. Dr. DeGangi was the therapist for these groups. Dr. Nemiroff has come to these transcripts for the first time. We hope that our own dialogues about the material facilitate the reader's own inner dialogue about understanding group process with children, and the interaction of regulatory and psychoanalytic factors.

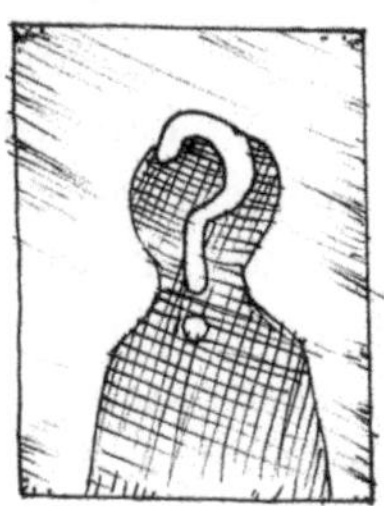

CHAPTER 1
"Mirror, Mirror on the Wall: Who Is the Smartest, Cleverest, Cutest, and Bravest of Them All?"
Children Talk about Identity

The First Letter: Being Invisible

The first letter in this section sets the stage for children to describe their problems to one another and asking others for advice. It is written to help children understand the importance of privacy and confidentiality and that asking for advice is respected. The voice of the child in the first letter demonstrates insight into his predicament while yet portraying vulnerability. The child in the letter expresses how alone he feels with this problem, teetering on the precipice of asking for help and shutting down from the world. The child presents an open invitation to other children to join him. The letter will hopefully resonate to any child who feels like a misfit and who yearns to belong to a group. All the letters have a boys' version and a girls' version. Occasionally the wording of the two versions is slightly different.

Feeling invisible is not uncommon among children with social problems. Latency-aged children often talk about hiding their "real self" from others. Some children fear that peers might ostracize them if only they knew the "real person" that lies within. Often a goal of therapy is to help children feel comfortable with who they really are, and to learn how to convey personal authenticity. This lays the foundation for developing intimacy with others as they continue to develop.

Providing enough detail in a letter is important. Giving everyday examples of problems that children might confront helps to make them feel realistic to the listener. However, there is a risk: some group members who provide advice may over-focus on the examples in the letter and thus overlook or defensively avoid addressing the true problem presented in the letter. The therapist's job, therefore, is to reframe the child's problem and gently facilitate the group process toward addressing the letter-writer's true problem. An integral part of the problem-solving process is being able to view the problem with clarity and perspective.

Dear Kids' Club,

I heard that this is your first group of the year. I am a 10 year old boy (girl) in fifth grade and wanted to write to you about something that I can't tell anybody about. Since you don't know me at all, it is easier for me to say my problem. Georgia will tell me what you think I should do. I don't think that anyone cares what I am thinking or feeling inside. Whenever I start to tell people what I feel, they glaze over, look bored, and change the topic. I feel that I don't count. No one cares and I feel invisible. I am giving up on trying to share anything I feel. I can't tell you how lonely and depressing this is.

I don't have any real friends, and even kids I see at school pass me over. You would think I was really hideous to look at, but I am average looking like everyone else. I don't smell bad, I take care of myself, and I dress nicely. I don't get it. Here is another example. When we play soccer and they are passing the ball on the field, I yell, "I'm wide open. I'm ready" and they completely ignore me. I am not a dud in sports so that doesn't explain it. I feel like giving up on trying to reach out anymore. How can I get other kids to listen to me when I share what I am thinking or feeling? Does anyone in your group feel that they don't matter to anyone and don't count? How can I get kids to notice me and want to be my friend? I am getting desperate.

Signed,
Thomas, The Invisible Boy
(Christina in girl's version)

MN: As I was listening to this letter, I felt myself sinking. The letter-writer's poignancy and depression are palpable, and yet he is not shut-down or lost in a glaze of withdrawal. There's definitely something alive, like a beating heart that hurts.

GD: In writing this letter, I wanted to convey a child who had not completely given up, but who still feels invisible to others. He is overlooked for no obvious reason. This is the kind of child who is likely to present affect that is disengaging to other children, a child who unwittingly does not evoke an inviting response from others. Everything else is going well for this child. He is constitutionally intact, but has social challenges.

MN: On one level, he's not befuddled about himself. He said that he was good at this or good at that. He isn't funny looking. He has an ability to reflect, which a lot of kids don't necessarily have.

GD: In a number of the letters that I have written for this series the child is insightful, because I wanted the kids in the groups to self-reflect. It's a model I hoped the children would learn to follow.

Boys' Group #1

Henry: I had this problem happen to me once. Let someone else talk first.

GD: Henry is a very shy and anxious boy who happens to be a lot like Thomas in the letter. He is often overlooked at school by his peers. What sets him apart the most is his affect which can be flat and disengaged.

MN: In terms of group process, Henry is presenting to the group a variation of the letter writer's problem. He's acting-out his problem. He sets out his affinity with the letter-writer and then stops, turning his visibility into invisibility. But you won't let him.

Therapist: What about on the soccer field? He would like to get a chance for the ball.
Henry: The thing about that, they always pass to the good people because they score the points. You said you're not bad though. Try to find a position that you're good at like goalie. You get more credit if you save the ball.
Therapist: Maybe if he had a position like that, they could count on him and he would feel important. What about when people tune him out when he's talking?
Jacob: Walk around with a microphone and they would really hear him. I know, make a really high pitch sound so it will hurt their ears. They'll really notice that.

GD: Jacob was a lot like the comedian, Jerry Lewis. He turned every situation into a joke, pushing everyone until no one could stand to be around him. He was using bravado to minimize the problem.

Javier: I don't think that'll solve the problem.
Henry: Talk to them about stuff you like. Two or three people might like what you have to say. Not everyone is going to be your friend.

GD: Henry is a very lonely boy. He had no friends when he came to group. His mother told him that he was participating in an experiment with me. She said that he was helping me out by doing this experiment. He was going to do it for one semester only, but at the end of the fall, he said, "I like being here. These kids really understand me. This helps me out to feel understood." He saw through the experiment quite quickly. This letter is about a kid like him.
MN: From a prognostic view regarding healthy group process, that would suggest his potential to be a group "insight-leader."

Henry: If you find those people that are nice to you, then they could be your friends. They'll help you when you get a good relationship going.

MN: He used language that's mature.
GD: He did. He was a very smart child.
MN: The fact that his language was cerebral tells me that he was distancing himself from what he was feeling. He was touched, but he was trying to move it away and put it back on the non-existent Thomas rather than on himself. He even said at first that he has a problem like that in the past tense. He described pulling away from people and he had just recapitulated it in the group process.
GD: He was a very intelligent child who was interested in science and math and would distance himself at school. He got very good grades but isolated himself and lost himself in books. Although not diagnosed, Henry presented much like a child with Asperger's syndrome. He had very little relationship with family members. Even his mother setting up the group experience as an "experiment" was distancing.
MN: Her tactic didn't acknowledge his pain, and therefore participated in his distancing from others: "you only have to do this for a little while."
GD: Henry's mom had a hard time connecting to her child. Interestingly, Henry always sat right next to me and responded well when I smiled and touched him.
MN: What did he look like?

GD: He was a plain child who might have gone unnoticed. There was nothing about him that would compel you to look at him or want to approach and talk to him. Henry would frequently gaze away from the group. I had to draw him into the group process by structuring jobs for him to do and by interacting with him in a very personal way. He needed structure to know how to be in the group. It's interesting that Henry says "Go get a job, like the goalie."

MN: He chose something very difficult. A lot of kids don't want to be the goalie because it's too much area to cover. It's interesting that he would pick something that a child might actually fail at. The flip side, of course, is that goalie can also be a star position. The juxtaposition of failure and success is interesting. His judgment was off in the kind of way that children with Asperger's misread cues and misconstrue meaning.

Therapist: I was thinking about the comment that he said, "Their eyes glaze over." Another way to think of this is when you're listening to someone, what makes you feel bored? What makes you feel interested? Maybe they're getting bored because what he is talking about isn't very interesting.

Henry: I think I know. Cut down your sentences. Don't make them too long. Pause and break so that you can see if they're interested.

Therapist: So it's the way you talk, not just the topic.

Henry: It's very good to have a friend.

GD: Isn't that sad?

MN: His language is itself very interesting: the verbs switch. He talks in a cerebral way, then says "You can see if they're interested" in an implied future tense, and uses the verb "to see" in making connections with people. In our culture, interpersonal connection is a visual phenomenon at first. In other cultures, this is not true. So we as therapists also have to understand our patients' cultural backgrounds in order to "read" their communications.

GD: Henry was an American child. He would sit in group and gaze away. I had to orient him visually back to the group. He was willing to interact with me, talking directly to me rather than the other children. He was the kind of child you can picture as an adult, living life alone in a dark place, not engaged with anyone.

MN: Did he ever talk about the books he read? That's a solo activity and we might learn more about him through conversations about books.

GD: Yes. He would lose himself in his books. He liked checking out from life through the fantasy of his book.

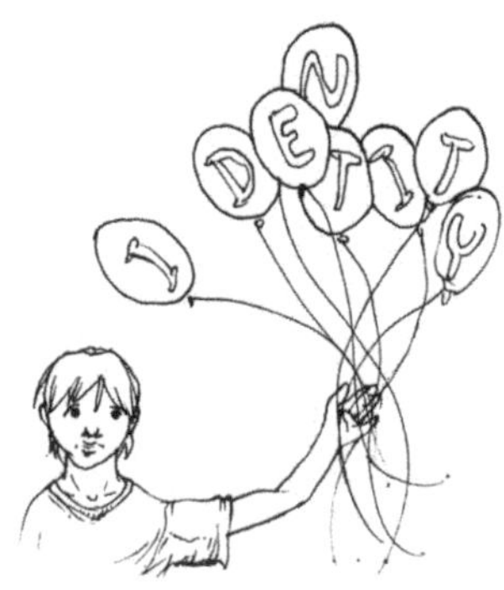

Girls' Group #1

Rosa: I think that you should be nice to others and treat others with respect.
Therapist: That's a good idea. Any other ideas what she could do when others ignore her?
Mallory: She should ask why she is being ignored by everyone and what's wrong with her.
Therapist: That's a great idea, Mallory, because she doesn't really know why she is being ignored. She thinks it could be anything. "Why are you passing me over?"

GD: I switched purposely to the child's voice to draw the girls into what the girl in the letter might be thinking.

Therapist: Anybody else have an idea? (No response from anyone in the room. Long pause.) Has anyone in this room ever felt this way?
Crystal: Nope.
Rosa: Sometimes I think no one cares about me and I feel very lonely inside.

GD: Rosa's comment, especially in group, was very powerful. She often did things that were obnoxious and inappropriate. Her responses to others were stereotyped and automated. She was often very self-centered, focusing on the immediacy of her needs like asking for the snack when someone was talking about something upsetting. There were times that she showed empathic failures that could be jolting. She frequently said things that were off-topic and self-absorbed, for example not tuning into a girl sitting next to her who might be crying or expressing severe distress. One girl had recently shared with the group that she had a serious medical condition that was progressing and how worried she was about her future. Rosa became very anxious; the only way she knew how to cope was to distance herself from the other child. Usually Rosa needed to be comforted herself—to ask for food in an urgent way, gobbling it up, asking for more or even wanting the snack off other children's plates. So for her to say "I feel very lonely inside" was very touching. However, her emotional attunement continued to turn on and off like a faucet.
MN: With her comment, she was not operating on pure need. Her impulse was properly ego-mediated. She was not being primitive. What happened?
GD: Perhaps she resonated to something in the letter.
MN: I'm trying to understand if she was resonating exclusively to the letter or also, for a change, to the reality of the other girls in the group?
GD: It's very hard to know because the other girls were shutting down as they heard this letter. I tried to voice for the child in the letter "Why are you passing me over?" to tune the group into the experience of the girl in the letter. Here's how it ends.

Therapist: So you really know how she feels.
Rosa: Don't worry, I'll be your friend.
Mallory: That's very sweet.

GD: In this particular session, Rosa showed us that she can be attached and present in the moment, even if it was fleeting and hard for her to sustain. Most of the time she feels programmed and reminds me of how some children with Asperger's syndrome are coached to say certain things in order to manage socially. But here, Rosa was speaking very much from the heart. There were tears in her eyes. I remember feeling a chill down my spine as I thought "Something got in there!"

MN: The letter got to her. The question: was it truly empathic? Did her comment have the poignancy of felt experience and of joining with the letter-writer when you heard her say it?

GD: It did at that moment. My usual experience of Rosa was that she turned away when other girls expressed heartfelt emotion. Rosa's own affect was very flat. Her eyes sometimes rolled upward which made her seem odd and disengaged. It was likely that she had a genetic syndrome because she looked quite odd. Whenever I spoke to her mother in the waiting room, I tried to relate incidents when Rosa was able to pull together a socially appropriate and empathic response. Whenever I brought up times when Rosa had difficulty connecting to other children (like the incident when Rosa could not tolerate hearing about the other child's medical illness), I suggested how Mrs. D. could talk with Rosa to help her with her own feelings about her friend and teach Rosa what she could say to her. Rosa goes to school with Amy, the girl with medical problems.

MN: Did the mother have the empathic capacity to follow through? So often a child's difficulty with empathy is based on early caregivers' problems with emotional attunement.

GD: The mother sometimes reacted abruptly to me. She would say something like, "Oh I know that Rosa has empathy! It is not a problem for her!" The mother's affect was somewhat similar to Rosa's—very stilted and formal. I'd worked with Rosa for four years at that time. Mom loved the group but I still didn't feel that I had a connection with her.

MN: It seems that they both have social difficulties and awkwardness. Rosa seems a very frightened child: frightened of her own affect and of her own vulnerability. When she's cruel, she pushes others away so that she doesn't have to experience her own vulnerability and her own sense of "not-all-rightness." Her mother may be frightened as well and feel emotionally vulnerable. Therefore, Rosa has a developmental dilemma in that she will grow up most likely identifying with a damaged maternal object, and one that may well be damaged in the same arena that Rosa is. If this pattern of identification should occur, it would serve to reinforce Rosa's already-existing problems.

GD: I do think that her mother walls off emotions in a similar pattern. There is also the problem for Rosa of what her home life was like for her. She was an only child and was left long hours to play computer games. I'd like to share something also about Rosa's fantasy life. Whenever we did open-ended art projects, Rosa often made constructions and a story line about how Frankenstein lived in the house with her. She created herself as the bride of Frankenstein.

MN: Did she understand that the Frankenstein monster was made from the body parts of others? What I mean is that the Frankenstein monster was a mismatched, unintegrated, collection of part objects.

GD: I think she must have. She was quite compelled by the story. She was a bit like a "piece-meal child." People had given her strategies—a laundry list of how to be with people, but she couldn't integrate them in a meaningful way.

MN: The best she could do with those strategies was to perform them. That is not enough.

GD: What seemed to be most effective was for me to work with Rosa in a relational manner. "You and me together in this moment, what each of us is feeling at this time and the meaning of our relationship to one another."

MN: You and I have spent most of our discussion on Rosa. I think this mirrors what happened with the group process. Perhaps they were as moved as you by Rosa's heartfelt disclosure.

Girls' Group #3

Deborah: For the first thing, write down your feelings on a piece of paper and read them. That might make you feel better. Because paper can't look bored or anything. Maybe she just needs to get her feelings out.

MN: It is so interesting that Deborah thought first of relating to a piece of paper rather than a person. Such an approach would reinforce one's invisibility. And yet, it is a partially adaptive way of expressing feelings. It should be a first step but Deborah seems to see it as the last step and it leaves her socially distanced.

GD: Deborah was very disconnected from people herself. She had Asperger's syndrome but unfortunately with a psychotic core. I also saw her in individual treatment. She sometimes heard voices that told her to do obsessive things. It wasn't just self-talk or the inner voice in the head. Schizophrenia and suicide ran in her family. Deborah lived in the world of books and was most comfortable enacting stories from her books. She could become quite self-absorbed in her own thoughts and, in the group, look lost in thought. I often needed to interrupt her to reorient her to the present moment. She was also a very private girl who had trouble disclosing anything personal. Her world of paper, pencils, and books were for her what people are for us.

MN: It's very troubling that she felt that people do not reinforce her emotionally. It leaves her alone in her mind with her voices. When she said "the paper can't look bored," I find that more troubling than I would from a more intact child because I don't actually know whether she experienced the paper as real. Her place within the group's process would be interesting.

GD: When she interacted in conversations, she was apt to go off in a soliloquy and quickly obsess over details that most people were not interested in. In working individually with her, I found it easier to gain emotional access, but we had to do a lot of story telling as a way of connecting with her feelings and in helping her understand her internal life.

MN: You had to rely on the technique of displacement, something we might do with a younger child.

GD: This next child was very complex. Gillian had cerebral palsy and walked clumsily. Her speech was very difficult to understand. She spoke slowly and stumbled over her words, as if she were talking with marbles in her mouth. She often had a lot to offer, but the other girls become impatient with her because of her speech. Usually they tuned her out after her first sentence or two, which resulted in Gillian not getting the positive feedback that she so desperately needed. She identified strongly with playing sports even though she was unable to compete with her peers in this way. Competition was a real trial for her and she often screamed at her younger brother who was well-wired, very competent, and gifted in many ways. So you will see from her response here how she presented herself to others in the face of these issues.

Gillian: Christina, I have a solution. When you're playing sports, because I love sports, just be in there and sooner or later the boys and girls will kick the ball near you. Then when it's wide open, you can go and kick it. You can do that. You can also tell a grown up that they're not passing the ball. The grown-up can say, "You need to pass the ball to all the people here."

Therapist: I was thinking, Gillian, that when you said to go forward and kick it, it helps prove to the other kids that she can do it. Is that what your idea was? (Gillian nods her head.)

MN: It's very sad that Gillian identified so strongly with the most visible thing that she was least able to do—sports. When this failed her, she seemed to be at a complete loss, and so she resorted to going to adults to fix it for her. She seemed to have little sense that she can be effective in the world. I would imagine that being in group therapy was hard for her, particularly when her verbal communication was also ineffective.

GD: Gillian has very few resources available to her. Her choice for games was to do two things—throw velcro balls at the dart board on my wall or to play Yahtzee™ poker. Nothing else interested her. When the group was involved in any activity whether it was a game, drawing, acting, role playing, or constructing something together, Gillian quickly disengaged and tended to roam my room unless I structured how she might respond to the group process.

GD: The next girl who spoke was a child with fetal alcohol syndrome and who was adopted from Russia. She was extremely impulsive, easily agitated, and self-centered. Now and then she could turn on the switch and say something relevant to the situation.

Alexis: Well, you could write a letter to the teacher and talk to him or her about it and maybe get over the fear if you have one.

MN: Her response shows that she had empathic difficulty with the feelings of the letter-writer. Her words were: "the fear if you have one." She was probably a child who disconnected from her internal life and was driven by impulse.

Deborah: Mine isn't really an idea, but it's something that happened to me. Last year in Hebrew class and every time I had P.E., no one ever passed the ball to me not even once and I felt really really bad. I was going to tell the teacher but I never got the nerve to do it. I didn't mind because I stink at sports.

MN: She merged two ideas together that are dys-synchronous—Hebrew and P.E. class. That tells us something about the way her mind works.

GD: For Deborah to think through a logical sequence of what actually happened and how she and others felt was very challenging. You can see her stumbling block—not being able to get up the nerve to ask for help and articulate what bothered her, and to test out her hypothesis of what was happening to her.

MN: She dismissed her feelings quickly. Saying that she stinks at sports was an easy excuse to avoid bringing her feelings of exclusion into the group. She used language that suggests that she participates in her own exclusion/invisibility.

GD: Deborah and many of the girls in this group required me to bring myself into the situation so that the topic would become more personal for them.

Therapist: Deborah, I know exactly how you feel because I was always the last one picked.
Deborah: This girl, Hannah, told me that people talked about me behind my back and said that I was terrible at sports.

GD: Her response here told me that she actually was aware of how others felt about her. I think that her behavioral pattern was to give up trying to connect with others, then turn to her internal world. She was hard to reach out to.
MN: She was locked so much inside herself. Finding the key would be difficult.

Maya: When I was at camp we had one activity and I chose soccer. I was the youngest and nobody passed the ball to me. I kept stealing the ball from them and gave it a shot. By the end, the counselor made sure everyone passed the ball to me. They thought I couldn't do it and didn't give me a chance.
Therapist: This will help Christina, to hear that she has company, that other kids have the same problem.

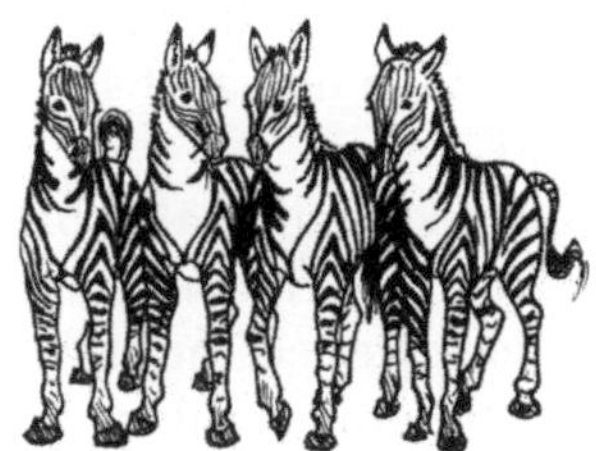

Girls' Group #5

Brooke: OK. How do I start?
Brittany: Well you could talk so that other people will hear you.
Therapist: Maybe that's part of her problem. She talks too softly.
Brittany: You could try talking to them and try making friends with them or find some other kids.

MN: This was a higher functioning group. They already were aware of what the girl in the letter felt and what they might advise about her problem.

Jacqueline: I don't know about this.

GD: When Jacqueline said this, she looked dazed and overwhelmed as if the girl in the letter was she.
MN: She experienced a loss of distance between the letter-writer and herself. That can be frightening.
GD: Jacqueline was a very compelling child who struggled constantly with anxiety and impulsivity. She was very curious and adventurous, but couldn't understand the nuances of situations and frequently ended up in a lot of trouble. She was ostracized almost daily by other kids as well as reprimanded by adults. She ends up feeling alone and misunderstood.
MN: That's very sad. It shows the complexities of how children feel when they are "invisible" to others. It is very important to uncover what lies under those feelings. It's not enough just to label feelings.
GD: The next child to speak was Brooke, a highly narcissistic child who was not well liked by the other children in the group. She frequently acted as if she had all the answers.

MN: A distancing defense that works in the short-run but actually is self-excluding; invisibility-making.

Brooke: Talk to a teacher about the soccer field. Ask the coach or PE teacher, "Coach, I need some help to get some people to pass the ball to me." Next time it might help. Try that.

MN: She's trying to wrap this up quickly. I think she's defending against the pain that the letter evokes in her. But you help her stay with it. A great example of the intrepid but respectful group therapist.

Therapist: That's a great idea. If she gets the ball they might see her talent with the ball. She asked if anyone knows how she feels. Anyone here? Look at this—three girls have raised their hands in here.

Brooke: We could all take the microphone and tell her, "We know how you feel!"

GD: I was amazed that Brooke was able to relate to the feelings that the letter evoked. As you mentioned, Brooke usually distanced herself, acting as if she was above any problems. For most of the time that she was in group, she would state, "I don't have any problems!"

MN: I think that the "being overlooked" quality of the letter-writer touched her own feelings of invisibility. Your description of her makes it clear that she only saw herself and that others don't see her. The problem was reciprocal: she could only see herself and therefore the group could not see her.

Nadia: Christina, I know how you feel because no one passed me the ball and I was really left out.

GD: Nadia, an anxious and shy girl, was overlooked at school and at home. The only way she could get attention was to mess up her bedroom, pull clothes out and strew them everywhere. Then her mother would pay attention by coming in and yell at her. Nadia also lacked the language skills to know how to talk to others. She was in a chronic state of being left out in life.

MN: Her language difficulties verbally trapped inside herself to such a large extent that she felt the need to rely on unacceptable-but-attention-getting behaviors. She stands to gain a lot from group in learning about the effect of behavior on others.

Therapist: Nadia, Christina will really appreciate what you just said.

Brittany: I know how you feel because I had a friend disappoint me once that she had another friend who was going to be her best friend, not me.

Brooke: Some of my friends at school don't include me because I have ADHD.

GD: Again I was quite surprised to hear Brooke relating to the girl in the letter. This was a huge opening for her to acknowledge any vulnerability in the group.

Jacqueline: What do I say?

GD: I was left feeling very sad from what Jacqueline says here. She is without words to express the sadness she might have been feeling. Jacqueline is often excluded, but because of her oddness.

MN: She does sound befuddled, but on the other hand, even "I don't know what to say" is an expression of feeling and therefore an act of communication.

Sometimes we don't credit such statements as having meaning. I'm glad she was able even to express her inability to respond.

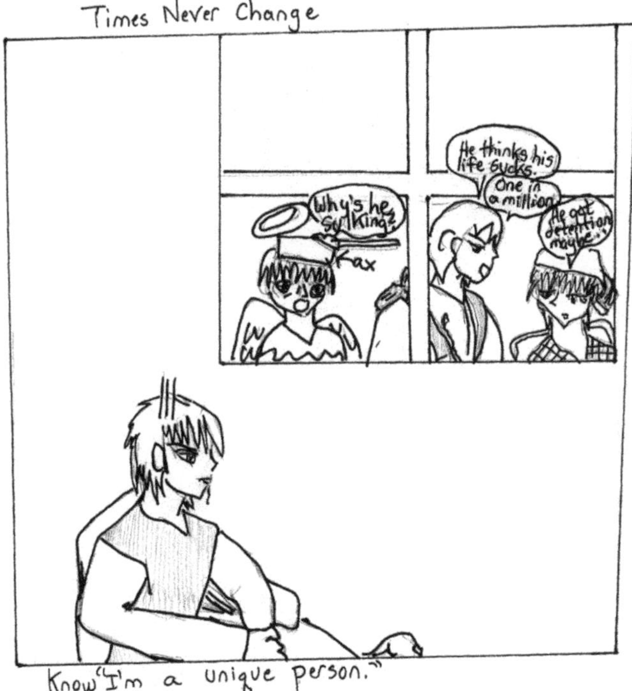
Times Never Change
Why's he sulking?
He thinks his life sucks.
One in a million.
He got detention maybe...
Know "I'm a unique person."

Suggested Activities

The following activity is designed to help children share features of their identity with one another in a safe way. Each child can fill out a handout with the following questions on it. When finished, all the group members can share what they wrote, or the group leader can read off the responses and ask the children to guess who wrote it.

1. What are some things that you like about yourself?
2. What are some things that you would like to change about yourself?
3. What problems do you have with friends and family members?
4. Do you ever have bad moods, get angry, get sad or depressed, or feel out of control? Circle which ones apply to you. Tell an example of what happens to you.
5. Do you ever feel stressed and overwhelmed? What makes you feel stressed?

References

Gemelli, R. (1996). *Normal child and adolescent development.* Washington, DC: American Psychiatric Press.

Leiberg, S., & Anders, S. (2006). The multiple facets of empathy: A survey of theory and evidence. In S. Anders, G. Ende, M. Junghofer, J. Kissler, and D. Wildgruber (Eds.), *Understanding emotions* (pp. 419–440). The Netherlands: Elsevier.

CHAPTER 2
The Square Peg in a Round Hole

This letter focuses on the child who worries about competence. Many children with learning or developmental challenges begin to notice in latency age years that they struggle to keep up with peers in academics, sports, and play activities. They may notice that their parents and friends find it difficult to engage with them in conversation or play because of the developmental problems that they experience. Some children may be passed over by peers because they are slow in sports, cannot keep up with a conversational exchange, or are limited in their play repertoire. Children like these may feel overwhelmed with daily life, with simply keeping up with everyday expectations such as getting up and out the door to school, with doing chores, arranging play dates, or thinking of things to do when they feel bored. They experience a growing awareness that something is wrong with them, that they are different, and that things do not come so easily for them as for other kids their age (Barkley, 1997). Comparisons to peers are made inadvertently by teachers, parents, and classmates. Gradually the perceptive children begin to see that they are minimized or overlooked. As they develop the capacity for mindfulness, they register others' facial expressions of frustration or boredom with them. In some cases, these children may become aware that their parents are dissatisfied with them, to the point of expressing disappointment in their child's continual struggle to learn or "get with the program" (Sroufe, Egeland, Carlson, & Collins, 2005). This letter reflects some of these issues and the emotional struggles that develop when such a child feels incompetent.

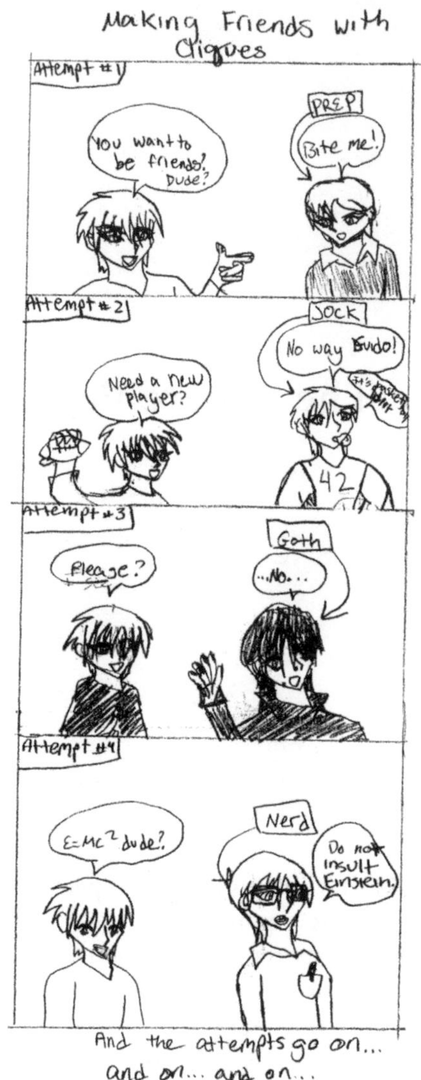
Making Friends with Cliques
Attempt #1
You want to be friends? Dude?
PREP
Bite me!
Attempt #2
Need a new player?
JOCK
No way Dude!
42
Attempt #3
Please?
Goth
...No...
Attempt #4
E=Mc² dude?
Nerd
Do not insult Einstein.
And the attempts go on... and on... and on...

Week 2
Dear Kids' Club,

I have a problem that I have a hard time admitting to anyone. I am not good at anything. I don't seem to do well at school and I flop in every hobby or after-school activity that I have tried. Here is what I stink at—math, science, writing, spelling, sports, art, music. You name it! If there is a kid who can't do it, it's me! The only thing that I did OK in this year was bowling and that was with the bumper pads. I even heard my mom and dad talking about me one night. They thought I had gone to bed but I was sitting at the top of the stairs listening to them. Now and then I have done this. My Mom said how disappointed she was in me, that I seemed to have no motivation and was a total goof-up. My Dad even said how he couldn't understand it because my younger sister was the big star in soccer, getting straight A's, and great in playing her flute. Yeah, yeah, yeah. She's the best! Gross me out! I'll tell you one more thing about this. I think that my mom is so bored being around me. Whenever we play games, she starts looking at her watch and yawning. I don't think I'm that boring to be around.

So, here's my question. What does a person do when they feel that they are a total flop at everything? I hate being me! I feel so stupid that I sometimes feel like smashing my head. Also, how can I get my mom and dad to not be so disappointed in me?

Signed,
Fred, the Failure
(Frannie in girl's version)

MN: The juxtaposition of his anger and his sense of being a failure makes my chest tighten. It certainly captures feeling misunderstood and worried about one's own abilities and competence. He sounds angry that he is unappreciated by his own parents and it segues into his own self-destructive behavior. I know youngsters like this all too well. They're banging their heads against the wall with self-loathing and anger turned onto oneself.

GD: I wanted to capture two sides of the coin in this letter—how devastated a child feels when things don't come easily to him as well as the disappointment and frustration that he perceives how his parents feel about him.

MN: A terrible discovery.

GD: Often parents inadvertently make comparisons to siblings or peers. In their interactions, the parent may become disengaged or bored, not knowing how to connect with their child. I often hear parents describe how hard it is for them when their child is unable to come up with play ideas or engages in repetitive play. But as the child reaches 8, 9, or 10 years of age, he becomes aware of his difficulties. The problem becomes compounded by the anger he feels at his plight.

MN: One thing we need to remember is that this is written from the child's point of view and it's his experience. He sees that he's not interesting to others. He is aware of his own despair or bewilderment in not knowing how to relate to others. He sees his parents as uninvolved and unable to connect with him. The resultant sense of isolation reinforces his loneliness and self-criticism. I worry about how youngsters like this will manage the internal and social pressures of adolescence, about whether there will be a growing alienation from others and/or a growing aggression that might get turned upon them.

GD: This letter also captures a problem of some children with learning disabilities who struggle with feeling competent in general. These children often have problems organizing social cues, gestures, and facial expressions that would give feedback to others. I was just thinking about a girl I see who is very flat in her affect and who works very hard at everything in her life. She gives such sparse feedback to others that other kids tune her out and exclude her. She feels that she is rejected and a failure. I wanted to capture the feelings of a child like this in the letter. However, the boy in this letter has enough gusto to fight back about his sister. His anger will help mobilize him to do something about his problem.

MN: He also has a sense of humor. Humor is almost always a good prognostic indicator.

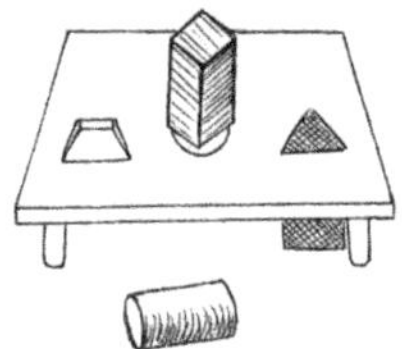

Girls' Group #1

Rosa: Practice makes perfect. Whenever I played basketball, I couldn't shoot baskets. The only thing I could do was dribbling. And I'm getting good at it. Shooting balls. Practice makes perfect.

GD: Rosa's language is very scripted.
MN: Yes. Was she a youngster with Asperger's syndrome, in which we see stereotyped language or some constitutional problems?
GD: She had a severe non-verbal learning disability.

Therapist: Other girls—have you ever had to work hard at something to get better?
Rosa: I'm good at diving too.
Therapist: What about Frannie's mom and dad being disappointed in her and her having this younger sister who is so good at everything? What about that problem?
Mallory: That's mean.
Therapist: What should she do?
Mallory: I don't know.

GD: Mallory was usually at a complete loss in a situation like this. She functioned as if she had a non-verbal learning disability, but in fact, her test scores showed that she didn't have this problem at all. She went to a small, private school. Without the support of that environment, she could not have functioned even at the level she was. She would be overwhelmed with anxiety and at a complete loss for understanding the most basic of social interactions.
MN: "That's mean" was an interesting comment. She was describing how others treated the letter-writer, especially the parents as intentionally hurtful. They're perceived as purposefully trying to be cruel when that's not what they were doing. From the letter there is no implication of parental intentionality. But Mallory's experience of it was of accusatory parents.
GD: Mallory was very concrete and immediately assumed that people were hurtful to her. She was the youngster who enjoyed tying nooses. It was her favorite thing to share in group for a long while. She looked like a very sweet girl, so there was a disconnect between her appealing outward appearance and her dark, destructive, internal emotional life. Her thinking process was to engage in persecutory fantasy, wanting to kill off the "persecutor" in retribution.

Abby: Always keep trying at it.

MN: This comment has a bromide quality to it. But at least Abby was trying to get some verbal group process going.

Therapist: Was there something in your life when you had to do that, when you got discouraged and you had to keep trying? (No response.)

MN: You were working really hard here to involve the girls with the painful material in the letter.

Therapist: I was noticing that the skeleton you drew today and brought for share is a very good skeleton. I imagine you had to practice a long time to get it so good.

GD: I was really trying to integrate and relate what they brought to the group to what is being talked about in the letter.

Abby: I actually looked at a picture and copied from that.
Rosa: I was bad at drawing and had to work hard at it.
Therapist: Let me ask you something. Does drawing ever make you feel better if you are sad or angry? Can you say something about that?

GD: Because it was hard to get the girls to think about the letter-writer's distress, I decided to focus on them and how they expressed feelings when they were distressed or overwhelmed.

Abby: She can draw how she is feeling.
Therapist: How do you draw your feelings?
Abby: I draw angry and sad.
Therapist: What would the anger look like? What color would it be?
Abby: Red.
Therapist: Does it have a shape?
Abby: I don't know.

MN: This conversational fragment demonstrates the growth of internal tension. Red is a hot color. In our culture, it is often associated with strong, often negatively intense, feeling.

GD: The only girl in this group who could acknowledge her anger was Rosa. The rest of the girls consistently looked flat and immobilized, unable to express their anger. When I was able to gain access to Abby, she talked about being teased mercilessly by the boys at school. She would be immobilized by these incidents and would take a long time to tell anyone that this was happening to her. She is the youngster who spoke very softly and had difficulty forming her thoughts into words. When she did speak, she frequently was overlooked and then she felt passed over. At the time, she had recently been saying, "No one listens to me and it makes me furious." But when she spoke of her anger, her affect did not match her words.

MN: Was she dissociating then?

GD: Not dissociating. It was as if she couldn't bring into her language the affective connection. Her language-learning disability was so profound that she lost the ability to describe her emotions.

MN: I mean the original definition of dissociation. Not the way we use the term now. It originally referred to the incongruence of what you're actually experiencing and the feeling that is attached to it. They can't come together in an integrated fashion. Here we have an example of the development of a specific defense as a function of constitutional problems. Both factors are at work, I think the intrapsychic and the constitutional problems. We need to take both factors into account in order to fully understand this youngster.

GD: This makes sense when we think about anxiety disorders. Abby felt mounting anxiety because she couldn't express what she felt internally.

MN: It's like Helen Keller. Trapped inside herself until helped to emerge and express herself. She reminds me of a girl who was so learning disabled that the only thing she could do competently was mazes. She couldn't narrate a story or understand the rules of a game. Her drawings were awful, but she would try. One time she had written something which nobody but her mother could read. She had, in unreadable fashion, written her Will. She was going to kill herself by jumping off the roof. Her Will told who would get which of her toys when she was dead. She had added, because she knew she was a burden to her parents: "All of you will feel better when I'm gone." What shifted her in treatment was a drawing she made one day. I was on the other side of the table and I was drawing too. She looked up and said, "You like me! You really like me!" (I did, very much.) Despite everything, there was somebody who could resonate to the person inside her very constitutionally damaged shell and see who was really in there.

GD: What a lovely story. Sometimes children need to express through drawings, music, or movement what is felt inside because there are no words for it. I followed this theme in my next discussion.

Therapist: Maybe it has different shapes depending on the anger. Perhaps Frannie could draw her feelings to help herself. Do you think Frannie should tell her mom that she feels she is a disappointment and that her sister is the favorite?

Mallory: Yes.

Therapist: How would she tell her mom? Like—"Mom I notice that you yawn and look bored when you are around me?"

Mallory: She should tell her without hesitation.

Rosa: I'm the only child so I get all the attention and praise in my family.

MN: Was that an escape from the affect?

GD: Yes, it was. Rosa departed to a self-centered place whenever she was overwhelmed.

MN: How did the group deal with that? She had just yanked the group off-course. The group was finally working with you here and then Rosa entered the discussion and disrupted the group process.

GD: They became frozen and returned to being hard to access. When Rosa would say these things, I felt like I had been hit with a stun gun. I had just gotten the group working and she yanked the group away from interacting with one another and toward her own egocentric world. There was a decided lack of empathy on her part. I was annoyed with her.

MN: It was a reenactment of what was in the letter. It was Frannie's situation in the letter. Rosa had made you disappointed in her.

GD: Exactly. I could feel my frustration at her, but instead of focusing on what Rosa had done, I kept my focus on the group and tried to bring it back to where we were.

Therapist: Well, Mallory and Abby both have brothers. Do you think she should tell her mom right away about this? If you started the sentence, what would it be—"Mom, I want you to know . . . ."

Mallory: But I never felt like that.

Therapist: Sometimes it's hard for kids to put themselves in other kids' shoes. I'm glad that you have never had this happen to you.

Rosa: Especially me.

MN: You over-rode this intrusion by Rosa and kept your focus on the group.

Therapist: You know what it tells me is that every one in this room has things that they feel good about.

GD: I tried to end it on a good note, but I was very aware of how painful this topic was for them. It was hard for them to speak about the devastation that someone might feel when others perceive her as incompetent.

MN: This letter was disruptive to a lot of these girls. They couldn't really deal with it at first. Then when they were finally working with you about their feelings and they were even attempting a little problem-solving, the process was disrupted again by Rosa. I wonder if the group was annoyed or relieved? Certainly Rosa's style of being in the group would become something to be worked with as time went by.

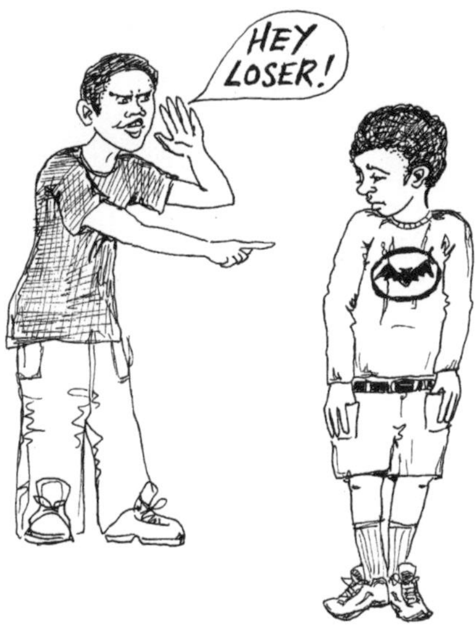

Suggested Activities

1. Each child in the group builds a diorama of a space where they would like to live. This place should be one that makes them feel very safe and allows them to be the person who they really are or wish to be. The base for the diorama can be a shoebox or a flat piece of cardboard. Found materials such as wood pieces, corks, corrugated paper, stones, pipe cleaners, and clay are ideal because of their open-ended nature. Children can build furniture, construct fences and windows, or a complete fantasy world of their own invention. This activity sometimes takes several weeks to finish.
2. Using an outline of the profile of a head, each child draws inside the different emotions that they experience. The "head map" can include anger, frustration, distress, anxiety, happiness, sadness, excitement, curiosity, creativity, boredom, and other emotions. It is helpful to have a list or a poster of emotions that children can refer to in helping them construct their "head map." They should create larger spaces in the "head map" for those emotions that take up more space. Use this activity to talk more about how the child's internal emotional life is experienced by them.

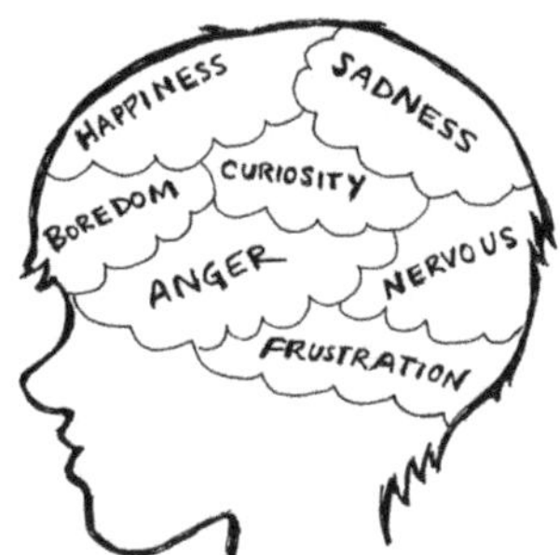

References

Barkley, R. A. (1997). *ADHD and the nature of self-control*. New York: Guilford Press.

Sroufe, L. A., Egeland, B., Carlson, E. A., & Collins, W. A. (2005). *The development of the person*. New York: Guilford Press.

CHAPTER 3

Jack Sprat Got too Fat, His Wife Got too Lean

The letter in this chapter reflects the complex feelings of rejection that a child experiences when others perceive his looks or body as not measuring up to prevailing standards. Many children with sensory integration disorder or other kinds of motor problems are clumsy and may look odd when running, climbing, or engaging in sports activities (Klass & Costello, 2003; Miller, 2006). Some children are born with genetic problems that make their face unusual-looking, a bit "out-of-sync." There are others still who experience low muscle tone and find that it takes a great deal of effort to move about in their spatial environment. The hypotonic child may opt for sedentary activities. Some children turn to eating because of a limited repertoire of leisure time activities. Food also provides comfort to the child who is anxious and distraught about his body. It serves as a source of comfort and nurturing, especially when nurturance may not be perceived as forthcoming from caregivers and peers.

As children mature, it is difficult for them to go from day-to-day unscathed, as people in their lives may compare how they look to how other children look. If the child does not have sufficient self-esteem, the damage to her ego can be profound and long lasting. As the child enters school, he or she begins to notice how other children look. As children take more interest in their own appearance, they sometimes make comments or communicate non-verbally how they perceive others' looks, both favorable and not so favorable.

Children whose self-esteem is more fragile may dislike their own looks enough to slip into full-fledged self-loathing. Internal self-rejection can run deep. Some children try to hide things about themselves out of shame and embarrassment. A child may weigh herself in secret many times a day. Another may pull out her hair along the neckline or bite her nails down to the quick. Some children may, sadly, turn to more harmful behaviors such as self-cutting. Self-cutting is often found on the upper arm, where it can be hidden. Sometimes it is on the lower arm, and occasionally it is on the thigh. The "child" who wrote the following letter speaks to all the children who understand this terribly dark place of self-loathing (Box, Copley, Magagna, & Smilansky, 1994).

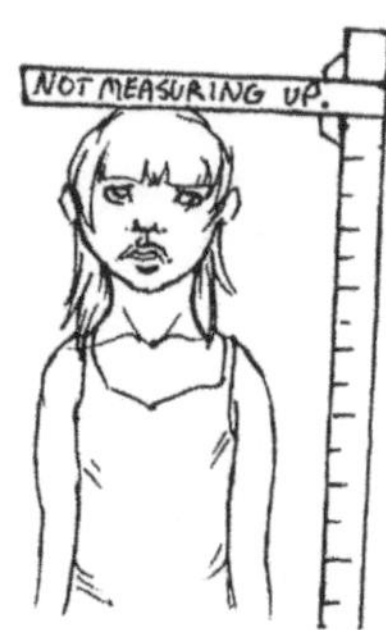

Dear Kids' Club,

I am very nervous to write this letter to you because my problem is one that is hugely embarrassing. I was born in a body that is completely funky. I don't really like the way my face looks. It is not an ugly face, but it is not a pleasing one. I am overweight and big for my age. When I run, people laugh at me, saying that I look like a big baby. I notice that when kids are talking and laughing with one another, they smile at each other but don't look at me. I wish that I could trade my entire body in for someone else's. I don't think there is anything I can do about this. It's the body I was born in. I get anxious when I think about this and start eating. I literally shovel the food in my mouth. That doesn't help the weight problem one bit and I know it. The other thing I want to mention is that I do something in secret. I am very nervous now to write this, but since you don't know me, I feel safe telling you. I sometimes think how much I hate myself and then I take a thumbtack or paper clip and try to scrape my arm to hurt myself. It makes me feel better—like an escape from it all. Please don't tell anyone about this, but give me any help that you can. Thank you.

Signed, Jonathan,
also known as "Fatso" and "Big Baby"
(Janice—girl's version)

GD: As I composed this letter, I tried to merge several children in my groups: one who had severe coordination problems and ran awkwardly like a "big baby," two who were born with dysmorphic facial features, and several others who would harm themselves because they hated themselves and/or their bodies.

MN: The process of transforming anger into self-loathing is very clear in this letter. It goes to the heart, his pain and self-loathing.

GD: I was hoping to capture the complexity of feelings that develops when body image issues emerge and there is little one can do to change certain things about one's body. For the child, then, the body gets confused with the Self. "I am Me" becomes "I am what my body looks like."

Girls' Group #3

GD: The first girl who spoke was the child with Asperger's syndrome. She was religious and sometimes reported that she heard voices.

Deborah: The kids when they laugh at her are just trying to get other kids to laugh. She should write down on paper all the things she feels. That's what I do when I'm angry.

Therapist: That's a great idea, Deborah. That's so much better than her hurting oneself.

Deborah: Don't let anyone know that you wrote the paper, write your feelings, then rip it up and scrunch it away.

MN: Writing down what she felt inside is a good release of the feeling, but nobody received the information. So she was still alone. And just in case you didn't understand, she repeated "I have my feeling and I'm going to get it out of me in some way. Nobody else will know about it." It ultimately left her very alone. I like this comment for teaching purposes because it demonstrates how our patients really do want to be understood. If we don't understand something, they'll often keep telling us until we get it right. This happens throughout the childhood age span, from pre-schoolers to adolescents.

GD: Scrunching the paper and throwing it away was a way for Deborah to destroy her feelings. In my response to Deborah, I decided to focus on the positive because she tended to obsess about things in a negative way. I wanted to try to disrupt this self-destructive process that was so ingrained in her.

Therapist: That's a great idea to let your feelings out. Is there anyone in here who doesn't like something about their body that they have thought about?

Alexis: Sometimes when I'm mad at myself, I just draw pictures of my anger.

MN: She wasn't only talking about her body. I think her self-directed general anger was being reflected here.

GD: Alexis was the physically tiny Russian adoptee with fetal alcohol effects. In the previous year she had become fascinated by her looks, sometimes showing up wearing makeup. It looked odd on such a young, small girl. When she responded to others, she often needed to focus on herself, but in the prior year she had begun to use art to "talk" about her feelings.

MN: Did she have the fetal alcohol syndrome features? The wide eyes, upturned nose, rubbery facial features, and diffuse learning difficulties?

GD: She had a pointy nose, long filtrum, wide spaced eyes, and a pinched look about her face. She loved receiving attention for being so physically small. She flaunted her smallness to others almost like an anorexic might do.

Therapist: Art is something that you really like, Alexis. So we have writing in a journal and drawing your anger in a picture as two ideas for Janice.

Gillian: Tell your teacher, your best friends if you have any of them, and your parents when you get home. Tell them what you're mad about.

Deborah: Something I don't like about my body is I'm too skinny and everyone says that to me. This girl is also probably too conscious about how she looks.

Gillian: Janice, I have cerebral palsy and I want you to know that sometimes I can't run right, or kids don't understand the way I talk. I try to ignore what other kids say to me.

GD: Gillian had never said to others before that she had cerebral palsy. She had tried to sweep that under the carpet because she was ashamed of it even though it was very obvious. I was so proud of her to open this door to others.

Therapist: That is so powerful what you just shared.

Ashley: I have this problem at school where these kids told my friend—I don't want to be your friend and if you are still friends with her, then we won't play with you at all. They would say, I want to be with you and you and you, but not you (to my friend). I had to tell them that I was going to stay her friend regardless and they have shut me out as their friend because I chose this girl. They don't like me because of this.

GD: She's departed from the letter to put her own problem in here, but I considered that this would happen in staging the Dear Kids' Club letters. I had hoped that

Gillian would have received some support but the girls didn't do that. But since I wanted them to bring themselves to the process and anything that might be accessed was fair game, I decided to let it go.

MN: Ashley was describing behavior that we hear about more from girls. Girls do this to each other much more than boys do. I don't know why. Ashley had a handle on this problem, the social morality of it. I notice that nobody was touching the cutting issue.

GD: That's right; no one wanted to discuss it, or, no one could address it. I chose not to bring it up myself. These girls might have been too young to be thinking of turning hatred inward to physical self-harm. The idea of cutting may have been too frightening.

Therapist: I think that Ashley is also telling us that finding a friend to be with you who can stand up for you is very important.

Deborah: This girl in my class is from Pakistan and people say she doesn't talk. She is very skinny and they tease her a lot.

GD: They ended with this comment—"someone we know who is like this, but it's not me with this problem."

MN: Deborah was responding to the process. She was filling in with a detail. It was more organized than some of the others of this group's responses. Bringing up the cutting with them would have been too provocative. They stayed away from the extreme of self-loathing.

GD: Gillian and Deborah held quite a bit of self-loathing for the group. In their individual therapy with me they would bring it up quite frequently.

MN: There was a decided progression in this session. The girls moved from giving concrete advice, to talking about their bodies, their own loneliness, and by implication of omission, the over-charged quality of self-harm.

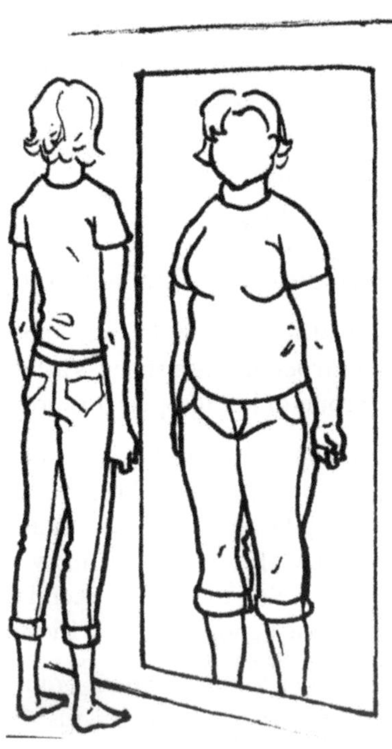

Boys' Group #3

GD: The first boy who spoke, Justin, had severe Asperger's syndrome. When I first began working with him, his language was word salad with no real meaning.

Justin: There is a misproportion of Fatso. The numbers make a misproportion known as Fatso. Control your anxiety and then you won't feel bad. Do some other things, like exercise, but not so much that you can't keep up with your homework. And I suggest that you eat good healthy foods. If you can get the weight problem down, and continue to be yourself. And I suggest that you not push the pin prick into your arm. Try to keep away from the refrigerator.

MN: It is interesting that the youngster with Asperger's syndrome was able to address the self-harm. Unless he was not as disturbed by the material as the other boys in the group, because his reading of the feelings of other people was atypical.

GD: A consistent thing about Justin was that if he was over-stimulated by sensory stimulation or emotions, he would run from the room. Gradually he was becoming better able to stay in the room and tolerated things that were happening.

MN: Justin reminds me of another child, a boy with Asperger's that I saw for so long—14 years. At a very young age whenever he experienced or even perceived negative feelings, he would fall to the floor and his atonia would become exaggerated. It was as if he would lose his skeleton and fall in a heap. His parents would call it "doing spaghetti." That's what it looked like. Or like the witch in The Wizard of Oz who melted to nothing. He simply could not tolerate that negative kind of feeling.

GD: That's an interesting example of what happens to the child's body when he feels so distraught. As soon as Justin talked about the pin prick, he backed away and talked about the child's eating problem. He could mention the self-harm but could go no farther.

Therapist: While he's losing weight, kids are still going to call him Fatso. So what should he do?

Nate: Call everyone else Fatso.

GD: Nate was a lovable child with ADHD, so that comment suited him.

MN: And it showed an endeAaronng capacity for humor.

GD: The next boy, Oliver, was a child with dark thoughts and real self-loathing.

Oliver: Don't say a thing! I want to suggest that you jump the gun and kill yourself. But if you do that, buy yourself a pair of Nikes. Jump off a bridge. Get out your Nikes!

GD: I worried a great deal about this boy because of his suicidal ideation. What was interesting was that he never disclosed these thoughts during his individual therapy, but in group he could safely bring them up. The Dear Kids' Club letters helped him.

MN: This is an example of productive group process. The Asperger's boy immediately picked up on the self-destruction theme. The boys were managing to work with this. But Oliver was a rather vulnerable youngster and he had inadequate defenses to prevent the self-loathing. He was drawn to it in the letter and in the group discussion. There was a bit of humor in his response but its mordancy worries me.

Jamie: Eat vegetables and meat. Don't eat anything bad for yourself for 3 years.

Oliver: Buy a pair of Nikes!
Therapist: It sounds like you would want to escape in a big way. The thought of feeling this way is so overwhelming to you. Can you tell me more, Oliver?
Oliver: My parents tell me that I am a genius, that I am by far the smartest person in the family. You can't have friends if you're that smart. I admire my brother who says stupid things and can be funny. It's hopeless for me. I can't be that way and I will never be able to change the way I think.

GD: That was a source of pain—being that intelligent.
MN: We see that in exceptionally intelligent kids: the ability to relate to others is compromised because they're very cerebral or cognitively so far ahead of everyone else that no one can relate to them, nor they to other people. They are alone. It can be sad to be "cursed" with such intelligence in terms of the social relatedness. Adults, including therapists, to lose sight of the fact that an exceptionally intelligence child is still emotionally a child.
GD: I often would say to Oliver's mother in private, "He will be fine when he gets to college and he can mingle with graduate-level students who are smart like he is, but we've got to get him there." I was very worried that he might harm himself before he gets there.
MN: I share your worry. One child I knew who was like this called me up when he got to college. He was extremely bright, a social isolate before college. Once he got to college and found other kids who were just like him, he said, "Marc, I'm not weird anymore. There are other people who are just like me here."

Therapist: Maybe you can't change your smartness, but you can change the way you feel. Instead of running away and escaping from your feelings, you can talk about it. I hope you know that we are here to help you. (No response.)
Therapist: I want to bring up that for boys and girls it's different. And for boys, it's not OK to cry. He could say, "It really hurts my feelings that you call me Fatso." but then he goes home and deals with it privately. Do any of you have sad feelings and are nervous to express them. Like if a pet dies, or something disappointing happens.
Jamie: Sometimes my pet stayed away for a day. He was hiding under the fence.

GD: That comment also made me feel really sad.
MN: Corey's wistful description of the sadness of loss is very touching. He's attending to the heaviness in the letter, rather than the self-loathing.
GD: Often boys don't have the venues that girls have for expressing these kinds of feelings. I was thinking about the hiding—what his pet did, and what these boys might do with their feelings.
MN: Corey had a bit of a touch of the poet about him. This was also unacceptable for a boy.
GD: He was a boy who in another year began identifying strongly with Goth. He would appear in wristbands, all in black, and even dyed his hair black. He did that to escape from social demands to keep up a certain image and instead to claim a unique identity that set him apart from others in a highly visible way.
MN: This session has progressed from mention of self-harm, to more alarming identification with the feelings of self-harm of the letter-writer, to feelings of sadness and loss, and isolation. The group started with the most difficult feeling and moved back to still-difficult but less threatening material.

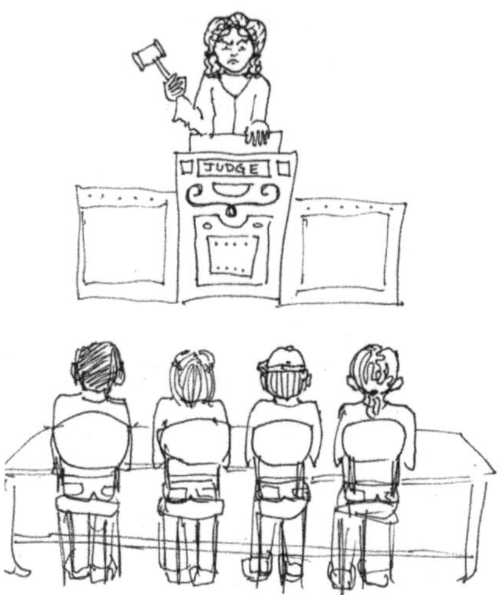

Boys' Group #1

Duncan: Is this really a real person? Oh dear! (Rapping microphone) Testing, testing.

MN: This is a great example of stereotypical boy-style avoidance. He started with a maneuver designed to express his worry that the letter-writer might be a real person, suggesting that Duncan identified with some of the feelings in the letter. He then worried whether (a) he could be heard if he should let out what he feels, and (b) he was "testing" whether anyone would be listening.

Duncan: Well—I do need to say that that's really disappointing for you that everyone is treating you so shabby and also, I just want to say that if I do tell anyone, you can punch me in the face.

GD: We've talked a lot about confidentiality and keeping things private. He got the message.

Therapist: He has your word. You're an honorable guy.

Duncan: And—when you said in your letter that you scrape yourself, there are some kids at my school that hit themselves and it makes them feel better.

GD: They were able to go directly to the issue of self-harm.

MN: Duncan's first comment in this session had to do with being punched by someone else, but nevertheless of being hurt. Was Duncan telling you that he understood how being physically hurt by someone or harming oneself makes some people feel better. Did he understand the relief of self-harm that certain people experience?

GD: Duncan had a chronic problem of picking on himself, pulling on his ears, to the point that he would fold his ears in horrible positions. I would ask him, "Doesn't that hurt you?" He had such an under-reactive nervous system that he didn't feel pain like most people. You wonder how much that was a factor as well.

MN: So in terms of this session, the very first comment was about hurting oneself. It was raised by a youngster with a constitutionally high-pain threshold. But he did select out from the letter the issue of hurting oneself. This is a dramatic beginning to the group session.

Javier: I do that, and it doesn't make me feel better. But I do it when I do a really stupid, obvious mistake, like in math. In the first test this year, I somehow subtracted 7 from 23 and came up with 15, which is really stupid. I know that 7 from 23 does not equal 15, but is 16.

MN: Despite his disavowal, I think Javier was indeed describing how self-punishment helps him feel better because it was a way of discharging his internal tension when he experienced himself as stupid. He's following Duncan's lead in the discussion.

Therapist: But you were so mad that you walloped your head?

Javier: And this is what we call a careless error or a stupid math mistake. They mean the same thing and you can't get rid of them. Even our math teachers do them every once in a while.

Therapist: You don't see them walloping their head.

Javier: Thanks for that.

GD: He said that with sarcasm in his voice.

MN: The sarcasm—what do we make of that? Was he rejecting what you were doing? Did he see you as critical? What was his proneness to narcissistic injury?

GD: In general, Javier's obsessiveness and perfectionism would prevail and he could get obsessionally stuck in these ways of thinking. I think that I didn't tune into his concern at the moment and, instead, I was staying with the theme of the letter. He was angry with me.

MN: I think he took your comment—"You don't see them walloping their head" as an empathic failure. It was then that he got sarcastic.

GD: To let me know that I had hurt his feelings.

MN: The theme of being hurt had now become acted out within the group itself in a parallel process to the boys' real lives and concerns.

GD: I had wanted to try to bring in that everyone makes mistakes. Unfortunately, I did not articulate that clearly.

MN: It let us know how really sensitive he was to tone of voice, to what was going on interpersonally, almost hypervigilantly. He would have been an interesting bellwether for the group process, the one to watch when you couldn't get a read on the group.

GD: In additional to their psychodynamics, Javier and Justin were both so hypersensitive to sounds and emotions; both would run from the room whenever there was too much going on for them. Even normal laughter would send Javier or Justin bolting from the room. I had to give both boys earplugs so that I could keep them in the room. Javier was home-schooled. He couldn't tolerate being in a regular classroom because of the noise. With youngsters like this, it's hard to separate out what came first: the constitutional hypersensitivity or the psychodynamics.

MN: Are the intrapsychic factors wrapped around the primary constitutional problems and developed in response to them? Or are the intrapsychic factors primary and then incorporated into the already-existent constitutional difficulties? Can these two be unraveled? And, I think more importantly for the therapist, is it actually necessary to even attempt to unravel them? Perhaps it is more useful simply to see them as co-existing. On the other hand, it is possible that subtlety of psychological makeup might be lost.

GD: It's an ongoing therapist's dilemma.

MN: I'm raising it not because it has a solution, but because we are obligated to think about it. A useful response would change from patient to patient.

Duncan: Jonathan, I know how you feel. I went to this school from another school because kids there treated me the same as you. I'm not overweight. I'm actually a light weight, but I was treated pretty badly. Those kids that were being so nasty to me, I hope they die soon. I'm sorry to say something so horrible. But I feel that I have finally gotten my own revenge. I'm sorry to say something so nasty, but I do know how you feel.

Therapist: You're speaking from the heart, Duncan.

MN: Despite the content, Duncan's response is rather appealing to me because of its directness. Clearly this child with Asperger's had obviously been benefiting from treatment. He was actually demonstrating empathy with the letter-writer, showing a proper reading of another person's feelings.

GD: Both Javier and Duncan have Asperger's and have benefited a great deal from their therapies.

MN: I like this interchange because it gives the lie to the oft-held opinion that you can't do therapy with children who have Asperger's syndrome because it requires a relatedness they're incapable of. It's really not true.

Duncan: Also, (long breath) two of my siblings might know how you feel. It's sad. They've been pretty disappointed for a long time. They're really nice looking, but their father got killed. And (long breath), that's all.

GD: Duncan was the product of a second marriage. His mother was married to a man who was killed in a horrible car accident. Duncan is recalling this.

MN: And recalling it with accurate, appropriate feeling. Those long breaths were also empathic. There seems to have been something lovely about him.

GD: I was very attached to Duncan. He was a peculiar child. My visual memory of him is him sitting facing the corner of the room, folding his ears. These letters were the most successful way to gain access to him, more than any other therapy technique I ever did with him.

MN: Probably because the letters were from anonymous people and this both allowed him emotional distance as well as removed the urgency of having to respond spontaneously in the moment to a real person. The group process is itself very striking. We have the stereotype that can't express sad feelings, and this group directly addressed the material from the letter. These boys were talking directly about their feelings. And to each other. I think this is remarkable.

GD: And here it's a group with many children with Asperger's.

GD: Tyrone, who spoke next, was a very small boy for his age. He also was facially different-looking. He had had a brain tumor removed as a young boy. He had significant learning disabilities.

Tyrone: I have something to share. If it's bothering you, just tell the teacher or try to ignore it or pretend that it's someone else instead of you.

GD: He had to use that defense at school. He pulled away and hid.

MN: He spoke of using two defenses: internal flight/fight ("ignore it") and depersonalization ("pretend that it's someone else instead of you").

Therapist: Tyrone, did you have that experience?

Tyrone: When I was younger.
Therapist: How did you do that—pretend they weren't bothering you?
Tyrone: I did it for a long time and finally they stopped bothering me.
Javier: I'm afraid I can't help you on the weight thing. It sounds like you want to lose weight and you have developed a habit that you need to break. That's up to you. I see other kids saying that you run like a baby, but by any chance do you run better than them? If you do, then I would say that they are just jealous and want to make you feel bad. If you run faster than them, leave the way you run alone. You're already doing better than the rest of your class.

GD: That's a nice spin that he put on this.
MN: He was trying to make the boy feel better. It's touching. This was a group session in which the members truly functioned as a group. The boys were responding to what each other said to the phantom letter-writer, but they were also taking their cue from what other group members had said. They were listening to each other and so their comments have a flow.

Therapist: I think everyone here has been disappointed and upset. You can advise him (the letter-writer) what to do about that. There's also one kid in this room today who is very upset right now.
(Aaron was mad at his mother for making him do homework over again. He exploded into the waiting room and came into the group late as a result).
Aaron: I'm not talking about that.
Therapist: Are you ready to explode?
Aaron: Yes!
Therapist: You're letting me know to stay back.
Javier: We have nitroglycerin in this class today.

MN: That was a group-level comment. Javier was being the pulse of the group!

Therapist: Going back to our coach and referee (kids in group had rotating "jobs" each group), your advice to Aaron was to leave him alone in the waiting room. Let him have time. Do you agree that we should do that now?
Javier: One other thing about the teasing, Jonathan.

GD: He returned to the letter instead of speaking about, or to, Aaron.
MN: He left Aaron alone, following the emotional flow. Javier was quite sensitive, in the positive sense.

Javier: I had that problem. Most of the kids in my class. All boys, because the girls didn't do this. And one mistake I made was doing what they wanted me to do. It made it worse. The irritation levels and teasing went up. Why on heaven and earth did I do that? It was the dumbest thing I've ever done.
Therapist: What was it?
Javier: Embarrassment factor.

MN: Javier's verbal shorthand, his on-target pithy comments came from really thinking about himself.

Therapist: I'm thinking about kids getting challenged to do things. I double dare you to do ... Like, pull down someone's pants and run back here.
Tyrone: That happens at my school.

GD: Great group process! Listen to that conversation!

MN: This was really very charming. What do you think was in this letter that opened them up so that they could function this much on a feeling level? They were responding to the letter and they were responding to one another in a lovely way and with a range of emotions. There was humor; there was anger. There was true respect for each other's feelings. And, there was a real attempt to connect with what the letter-writer was feeling. This group did a very lovely piece of work.

GD: The letters got more process going in the group than if I had relied on the level of content that they usually brought to the group or activities. The rest of their group activity was predominately building things together or making electronic devices. This was the only way I could get them to talk about themselves.

MN: Perhaps because they were initially responding to a person who wasn't really in the room, except as the personification of the boys' own difficulties.

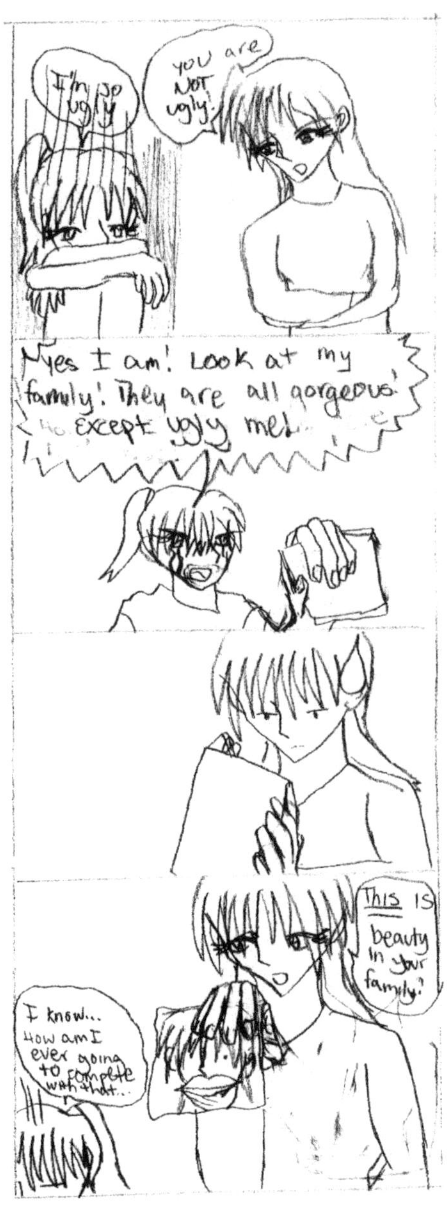
I'm so ugly
you are NOT ugly!
yes I am! Look at my family! They are all gorgeous! except ugly me!
This is beauty in your family?
I know... How am I ever going to complete with that...

Suggested Activity

Continue working on the diorama. Children can make soft clay figures of the characters they want to use in their diorama or they use playhouse dolls. The therapist should ask children to elaborate on who their character is (e.g., age, gender, occupation, talents, and personal attributes).

References

Box, S., Copley, B., Magagna, J., & Smilansky, E. M. (1994). *Crisis at adolescence*. Northvale, NJ: Jason Aronson Inc.

Klass, P., & Costello, E. (2003). *Quirky kids*. New York: Ballantine Books.

Miller, L. J. (2006). *Sensational kids*. New York: G.P. Putnam's Sons.

CHAPTER 4

From Butterfly to Moth

Adolescent Metamorphosis

Many factors affect identity formation. As a child matures, he becomes aware that other people may not know the "real me" inside him. A child, however, is not always sure whether he wants that "me" to be known. Most people share aspects of their "real selves" with those whom they most trust in the world. But, when a person's real, exposed, self is attacked by others, it can be very destructive. This letter addresses yet another aspect of the changing identity that is experienced by children in late latency—their interests change and their personalities begin the shift into a more mature self. Children may find that they are less interested in playing with dolls or action figures. They may not enjoy certain hobbies or activities that they once did. These changes occur at different rates for different children. Sometimes change frightens children. As a child changes, she may feel sad at "losing her old self," the one who had a zest for play and abandon. She doesn't yet understand, of course, the coherence of her development and that her "real self" is expanding rather than disappearing (Steinberg, 1999; Steinberg & Morris, 2001).

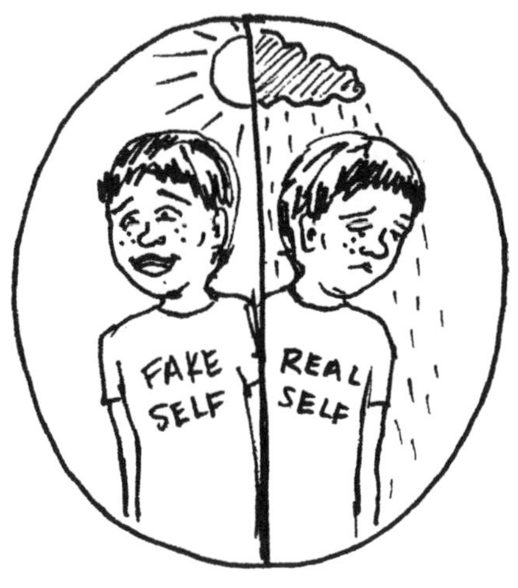

Dear Kids' Club,

The topic I am writing about is complicated and I hope that you will understand what I am talking about. When I was younger, I used to be really funny and talkative. I was great at computer games and liked playing outside, doing sports and exploring nature. I sometimes would make inventions from things I found outside, like making an insect world in a jar. When I got to be 11 years old, I started to change. The things that I used to like doing are different now. I suddenly became quieter and more thoughtful. I started reading a lot and making up stories in my head. Some of my friends that I liked before are ones that I don't really care to hang out with anymore. I find them a bit dull and goofy. It was like a switch went off inside me and I'm almost a different person than I used to be. I'm a little sad that I don't like doing the same things I did with friends. One of my friends asked me, "What's eating you? You hardly laugh anymore and you don't like exploring like we used to do." I miss doing our adventures too, but they don't really interest me anymore. I am different now. I want people to like me, but I am changing and I am trying to figure out who I am. I want to have friends who can understand me and know the real "me," not just people who *think* they know me. I guess that I am really wanting some friends who I can tell these things to who also feel the same way. I feel confused most of the time about who I am or who I am becoming. It's a bit scary. What is your advice about this?

Signed,
Charlie, the Confused Guy
(Chelsea in the girl's version)

GD: I wanted to capture the identity transition that often occurs in middle school.

MN: It coincides with the changes in the body and with youngsters feeling out of control. The "letter-writer" wonders "who am I" as a person, and may also be feeling internally "What is happening to me physically?" During the pre-adolescent growth spurt, the feet are too big and children bang into walls. The hormones are starting but are not in full force. Emotionally and physically, children have to "grow into" their bodies much like having to grow into their adult teeth when they emerge in an eight-year-old mouth not ready for them.

GD: In this stage of development, the face begins to look disproportionate and that little child look starts to change, sometimes dramatically. A look in the mirror may cause the child to pause and wonder, "Who is that person looking at me?"

MN: That's right. You need to grow into your physically changing self at the same time that you have to confront important psychological and emotional changes. That's what the letter-writer's wondering. "Who am I becoming?"

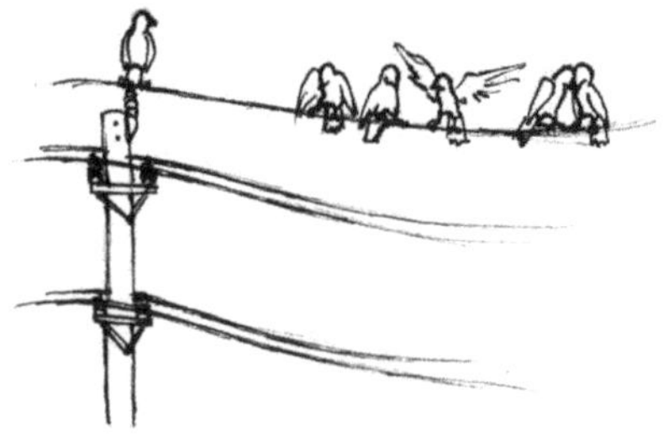

Boys' Group #3

Oliver: I am just like Charlie. I feel that I am so different from my friends and they can't possibly know what it's like inside me. (He looks at his cherry colored sweet drink.) It's a pool of blood and someone is going to jump inside!

GD: Isn't it interesting that the red-colored drink triggered this response in him? You and I have talked about the meaning of red and how it can elicit raw emotional material.

MN: Oliver's morbid pre-occupational tendencies certainly provoked an immediate morbid fantasy. He heard what the letter said, but he has used a visual cue to respond to it. The association was rather idiosyncratic. He was showing and telling you one of the ways that he felt different. And he expressed his morbid preoccupation with blood and intrusion in front of the other kids.

GD: Someone was going to jump inside the blood. He's talking about himself; it's a frightening and concerning image.

MN: Did anybody in the group respond to him, either in words or in body language?

GD: No. The group was flat. There was very little response to this letter in this particular group.

MN: Did the group's non-responsiveness have a flat, dead quality or was it paralyzed? Was there a sub-terranean energy present that was responsible for the defensive paralysis?

GD: I would say that it felt like paralysis and that was what I next responded to.

MN: This demonstrated the therapist's need to read truly beneath the surface, not just latent content, but also what is happening "underneath the manifest process" that is contributing to the group process.

Therapist: Sometimes feelings are so scary that they overwhelm us. Sometimes kids even joke around about something pretty serious that they feel inside. Is that what you're doing, Oliver? (No response.)

Justin: I have a suggestion for Charlie. You should take up some hobbies and join some clubs to meet some new kids who fit in with your new interests.

MN: Justin saved the group by getting practical.

Oliver: I know about changing. I used to be into Yugio™ cards big time and then the kids lost interest in that too. Fortunately for me, I had some of the new Magic™ cards and knew what they were all about when I went back to school this year. At least I could fit in that way.

MN: That's off topic in a way, somewhat tangential, because fitting in was not what this letter was about. It was about "Who am I?" Oliver, after having given the group a sense of his feeling that he's weird, chose to adopt with Justin's escape route: practical advice about fitting in. The group was moving far away from "Who am I?"

GD: They skirted the issue completely, but instead resonated to what was really on their minds.

MN: From a group dynamic framework, the group was working, but in defensive lockstep—monolithically. If you had asked something if there was about this letter that the boys didn't like, do you think they would have been able to work with that or would they still have been paralyzed by the content?

GD: I think they would have remained paralyzed, but that would have been a wonderful way for me to re-state the real issue.

Boys Group #1

Henry: This is called adolescence.
Therapist: What does that mean for you—going through adolescence? What do you understand about this change?
Henry: The frontal lobe of the brain is the part where it decides your personality and doesn't fully mature until you're 30. So it changes a lot from 10 to 16.
Therapist: Where did you learn that? That's important information.
Henry: Magazines outside.
Therapist: From my waiting room? (Therapist laughs) That's good. So Henry, what changes do you notice in yourself that you might want to share with Charlie?
Henry: I don't really notice anything.

MN: Dead end!
GD: Henry would learn everything through books rather than through interpersonal observation. He was also the boy who believed he was in the group because his mother told him that he was participating in an "experiment" and that he was helping me out. He had little self-awareness and would glean information about himself and the world through magazines in my waiting room and other places. This made it hard to know how accurate his information might have been.
MN: The stimulus letter was about a boy who has a lot of self-awareness, so it's interesting that Henry thought about the physiological aspect of change rather than the critical issue of "who am I? Who am I becoming?"
GD: This letter may have been too sophisticated for the group.
MN: Henry didn't know how to respond to it. He was aware of changes but he couldn't both personalize it and de-emotionalize it in order to tolerate it. I'm not sure that it was too sophisticated conceptually, but maybe it touched a frightening issue that this group couldn't articulate yet.

Therapist: Maybe you're not changing yet. Anyone else notice changes in themselves? That you like different things than you did a year ago? That you're different in their personality?
Tyrone: This is too hard to explain.
Therapist: Sometimes when you have these changes it can be embarrassing too. Maybe you don't like the changes or you don't want to share it.

MN: The group was getting a little stuck. Was it possibly too difficult for the boys to talk with a female therapist about this? Some boys are indeed more embarrassed with a female therapist at this time, but there are other boys who really do better and are less embarrassed and more open with a woman. Do you think the therapist gender was an important issue in this session?
GD: I think so and that's why I used the word "embarrassing." I chose, however, to continue and asked Tyrone about it.

Therapist: Is that part of it for you, Tyrone? The embarrassing part?
Tyrone: Yes.
Therapist: It's private.
Aaron: I'm hungrier and hungrier.
Duncan: If you keep on eating like that, you'll grow into a sumo wrestler.

MN: Aaron and Duncan were actually trying to retain the difficult issue of physical changes, but they did it with weight—with that which is publicly visible. Duncan, nevertheless, intimated through projection that he felt in some ways grotesque in appearance with the physical changes he was starting to experience.

Tyrone: At my school I see that people are hanging out with people from different genders.

MN: Here is a relevant shift, more approachable by the group.

Therapist: That's a difference too. Are any of you having the experience that Charlie is having where he wants different friends. A change in the group you hang out with—like being around girls instead of boys only.

Aaron: I like being around girls instead of boys. That's the way I am.

Therapist: How do you handle your friends if you've become more around girls?

Aaron: All of my friends are girls. None of my friends are boys. This happened at the beginning of this year.

MN: Did this have a confessional quality? Or some element of defensive bravado?

GD: Aaron had no friends except the boys in the group. He was trying here to present an image of himself as "the babe magnet." He'd like to be one, but he wasn't and he had such notable ADHD characteristics that he wouldn't be able to perceive this at all.

MN: Is this an aversion to boy stuff—away from sports?

GD: He has very little interest in boy things.

MN: Can we rule out sexual identity problems or am I extrapolating too far?

GD: I wondered if that was operating at the time, however, many children with learning disabilities like Aaron avoid sports because of poor coordination. Sometimes they are relieved when they reach adolescence and can become successful interpersonally by using conversational skills with peers.

MN: You would expect by age 11 more of a group of buddies—two or three same-gender friends. You see them in the malls going up and down the escalators, unable to keep their hands off each other.

GD: I think that Aaron's friends were more superficial to him. In my girls' groups, they talked about having a "boyfriend" when all the boys did was smiled at one of them. Aaron's idea of friendship was like that.

MN: Nevertheless, the group had a youngster who brought it back on-task. The issue started to get cerebrally laundered by becoming physiological in content. But then Tyrone brought it back to the feeling level. Was that a group role for Tyrone?

GD: Not at all. This letter must have elicited something in him. Tyrone was the boy who had a brain tumor when he was a preschooler. I wondered if he resonated to the part of the letter that addressed the issue of never fitting in.

Therapist: So you're saying that it's not a problem. How did you guys accomplish that? That's what Charlie is asking.

Javier: I accomplished it because my female friend is someone that everyone can't help but like. She's nice. She really likes to talk.

Therapist: It's easy to be around a person who has a lot to say as long as you get to say things too.

Javier: And she's very nice.

Henry: I haven't been attracted to girls at all. Nobody I know is interested in girls yet.

Therapist: That hasn't happened to you. Does it puzzle you that you're not interested in girls?

Aaron: It has for me when I decided to start dancing with girls. A big step for me.

MN: The group process got back on track.
GD: Something allowed it to re-orient itself. I think it was their moving away from their physical changes.

Henry: I'm in a special school and the social system is set up different.
Tyrone: There was a dance at my school last year.
Henry: Nobody dances at our school dances.
Therapist: Charlie, you may be interested in girls too, I hope this helps.

GD: I decided to close it off because this wasn't going anywhere.
MN: Javier said something interesting: "I accomplished this because my female friend is someone that everyone can't help but like." He wasn't talking about developing ways to be liked for whom he was or even to figure out who he was becoming. He was talking about doing it by proxy or by association. It's a form of avoidance.
GD: He would latch onto somebody else and would become the shadower, and then would get the attention by default.

Girls' Group #3

Kendra: Maybe you've gotten to be mature. When you get to a certain age, you mature a lot. When you're 13, you may be even more quiet. Maybe if you want to change so badly, you should. To start being funnier like you used to be.

GD: Kendra had a gender identity disorder. She came to group dressed like a boy.
MN: She implied that a person has more instrumentality in certain changes than she actually does. Physically you don't have any choice. Your interests could change, but you can't authentically force yourself into an interest that you don't have. There's little reason to suppress an interest that you have. Kendra was treating this as if she could have had much greater control over these things than she really could. She then undid it—"just go back to the way you used to be."
GD: She resisted being feminine, like the plague. She wore sports outfits and pulled her hair under a baseball cap. The therapist working with her individually would do "girl things" with her to help her become more comfortable with feminine activities. Her mother was not going to practice girl things with her. The therapist was hoping to help Kendra look a little more mainstream to fit in. Kendra was remarkably masculine, and at first glance, you would think, "That's a boy!" As she developed breasts, she went to baggier clothes to hide them. She also played in a baseball team as the only girl in the team. It was interesting that she said, "If you want to change that badly, you should," when she was so resistant to doing that herself. She had already decided what change she was going to adopt—her gender.

Gillian: If you're so sad about being quiet, talk to your mom and dad. "I'm getting to be a little quiet." You are a good person and I know that because a lot of people in this world are good people. If you can talk to your parents or whoever, just say, "I'm really sad and I feel lonely. Can you talk it through with me?" I'm usually quiet but I talked to this really good friend of mine and it really helped me. Now I'm a chatterbox.

Deborah: What you said about how you want to make up stories in your head, maybe you *can* make up stories. You could write them down. Right now I'm writing a story down. Write funny stories. Maybe inside you still are a little funny. You could write comedies and people could read them and realize that you still are funny. Talk to your friends about how you're changing and how you still want to be their friend.

Therapist: Has anybody in here experienced their friends changing on them?

Deborah: Not that I was maturing or anything, but my friend, Donna, she hardly plays with us anymore. She always plays with these different girls and we thought it was because she was getting popular. She said, though, that these girls hate her. Then one day she went back to playing with them.

MN: These youngsters got caught up in the social shifts that girls manifest at this age. It's a variation on pre-adolescent cliques. They were discussing social dynamics rather than identity change.

GD: This is a good example of how I got completely different responses from the boys and girls groups to the same letter. The boys went more to the heart of the topic—identity—whereas the girls got stuck on popularity. I think girls have a different dynamic than boys at this age.

MN: I agree. The social dynamics of popularity concern girls of this age, much more than boys.

GD: That boys' group was a generally high-functioning group, even though they were newly formed as a group. They had not yet developed group cohesion, and yet they were able to articulate issues on a higher level.

MN: So they were also speaking about the group process: what the pairings would be, what triangles would form, whom one might trust, whether they were going to be liked by this group, and so on.

GD: I wondered what their parents might be saying to them. Parents make a lot of comments about how their children should look and how they should act. I wondered if some of these comments reflected what parents said. "Just try this! Get outside and play. You'll feel better!"

Elizabeth: Friendship groups will change and that's because they're maturing. If you move to a new school like I did, then you become not friends with them anymore.

Kendra: Last year I moved to a new school in the middle of the year and I wasn't good with friends and stuff. Then I made friends because I talked to them. I got bad grades because I was paying more attention to making friends than schoolwork. This year I'm doing really good because I'm saying, "Work comes first."

MN: Kendra was still not attending to the issue of internal changes. It remained a matter of fitting in. She wasn't picking up the loneliness in the letter.

GD: I think that Ashley did that next.

Ashley: Three girls in my class (I have six girls counting me)—all they care about is what other people think of them. All they do is talk back to the teachers and tease everybody. I never liked them in the first place. I have one friend in the whole grade.

MN: She was getting closer to the issue, and in the process, over-riding Kendra.
GD: Yes. I seiqed what she said and suggested how alone one might feel during this time of identity shift.

Therapist: Is it lonely sometimes?
Gillian: If you are really lonely, maybe people think they're not playing with you or talking to you because you're quiet. You should back up your friend. Say, "Can you help me because I'm really lonely." People are really good citizens and help a lot. There are a lot of people who died and people who got hurt from the volcano eruption last Tuesday and they're helping each other to stop the Mount St. Helens eruption. 100 firemen and 20 policemen and people around the world helping you. So if you need someone to talk to, talk to your parents. They'll say, "Don't be afraid to talk." When I talk, I'm shy but I speak up. Then I say I'm good inside.

MN: Gillian said what really touched her—"I'm really lonely" and then went into the volcano, a classic symbol of internal tension, usually rage. So we can surmise from this that her internal tension and anger were prominent and possibly getting in her way. She couldn't really attend to "I'm changing in who I am and how do I make my way in the world now that I'm evolving." She was bringing in the stereotypical helpers. I do like, though, that she raised the issue of the volcano.
GD: I wondered if she was trying to say—"My loneliness is so big that it is like a volcano erupting. I need the help of 100 fireman and 20 policemen. That's how bad it is."
MN: So we can apply multiply meanings to the volcano. We do seem to have the inner tension of a volcano, but Gillian also used it to let us know that she felt lonely enough that she needed a lot of help. She was in so much distress. 100 fireman to cool her down and 20 policemen to keep her contained.

Kendra: Maybe if you don't have any friends now, when you're in class you can show kids at recess or PE how fast you are. Maybe they'll want to be your friend.
Ashley: There's this girl, but she was never my friend in the first place, but she's in my class. She's really shy and she doesn't like anything that I like so I'm really nice to her. She invites me over every day. And last time, I'd say, "Your dad is just about to be here to pick you up." 20 minutes later . . . .

GD: Ashley was alluding to the fact that she was being nice to this girl and the girl, in turn, was suffocating Ashley. Ashley was trying to avoid her. The good deed got punished.

Therapist: Ashley, you brought up something important. Some of the girls are getting a little snotty and image conscious.
Ashley: All they care about is being popular. One girl in the class is really my friend. Her goal in life is to be one of the more popular kids. But she is really a tomboy. I say, "Be yourself." The other kids don't like her.
Kendra: There's this one kid in my class—Laura. Last year she was trying to get all these cool clothes and stuff.

MN: She wasn't giving her full thought. She was assuming that everybody knew what she meant. Was the group process fading?
GD: Yes. I felt that the group process was fizzling out, so I responded . . . .

Therapist: She's changed this year?

Kendra: Yes.

MN: This group, in terms of its process, had questioned her and said, "I'm not sure I get it."

GD: No, they wouldn't or couldn't get it. Most of the kids in this group had ADHD. I wondered when they listened to the letter if they heard everything. What parts were they pulling out and attending to?

MN: A letter like this one has a lot in it. If you had asked them the question, "What do people think are the important parts of this letter," we might have been able to get a sense what everybody was keying into.

GD: That would be an excellent question to ask before saying, "What's your advice?"

MN: It would help focus the group. It is so hard for children with ADHD to be able to discern the most important bits of information from complex communications.

GD: The fact that I didn't get so much from this letter as some other ones suggested that the struggle of what's real and what's false might not be well articulated for these children yet. I think they needed more work on understanding, probably concretely, what it means to have an identity. The letter-writer's conceptualization of this may have been too sophisticated for them.

MN: Somehow, a few of the boys were closer to this particular letter. It should really be the other way around. Boys this age don't speak like they did, but your boys were managing to do it.

GD: I think having a female therapist in the room with boys was important even though I always co-led these boys groups with a male therapist. It brings us back to the point you made earlier about how we can't always predict which gender-match of therapist and child works best. Did this group do well simply because of who they were? Or because a female therapist was present? Or because a male therapist was present? Or because there was a gender-mix of therapists? We just don't know yet.

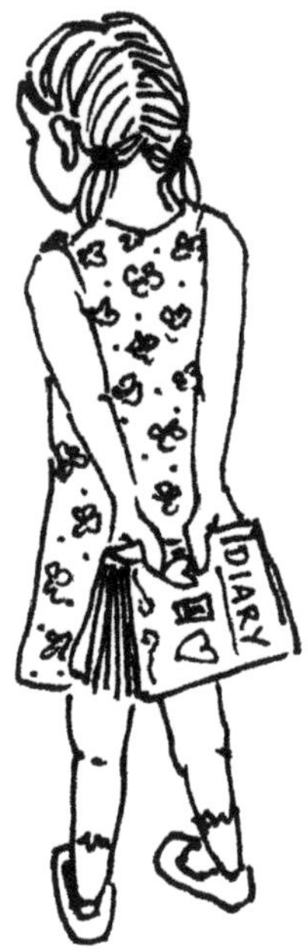

Suggested Activity

Using each child's diorama, ask the children to think of how they can fit each diorama into a city of their own making. Begin constructing a story line using the different characters that each child chose to be. Have each child describe whom she is, tell about their place, and plan a story that they will enact and film next week.

References

Steinberg, L. (1999). *Adolescence* (5th ed). New York: McGraw-Hill.

Steinberg, L., & Morris, A. S. (2001). Adolescent development. *Annual Review of Psychology, 52*, 83–110.

CHAPTER 5
Back-Stage or On-Stage

Our letter in this chapter regards a child with low self-esteem and who compensates for his insecurity by seeking to be the center of attention. This child demonstrates some of the typical behaviors and feelings that arise when a child chooses this mode of adaptation—showing off or bragging. People throughout their life need to feel validated and that they matter. Children usually receive validation of their essential worth from their parents. When this is insufficient for the child for some reason, or it is not forthcoming from the family, a youngster seeks it elsewhere, usually from peers. Some youngsters achieve this through appropriate sociability, others through achievements, still others from the development and sharing of common interests. However, some children resort to less adaptive approaches to the problem and, in seeking affirmation from others, actually push them away (Heaney & Israel, 2002; Greenspan, 1993).

Dear Kids' Club,

Hey, guys! I hear that you are having a lot of fun in your kids' club. I wish I could be in it with you, but I just can't. The reason why is I am in so many after-school activities. I am a little ashamed to tell anyone about my problem, but I figure that you kids are safe. I am a big show-off. Everything I do, I try to be the best there is and outdo whoever I am playing with. I think that I have a big competitive urge because I try to beat the other kids, be the winner, and then when I do win, I gloat about it and say how great I am. I can't control myself when I do this. If I lose, I feel like a complete idiot and worthless inside. Kids at school often say to me, "Everything is always about you. You are such a big show-off. All you do is talk about yourself." If someone tells a story about something they did that was great, the next thing I know, I am telling a story about how I did it better than them.

What do you think is really my problem? Is there anything I can do to stop doing this? I already have a reputation for showing off, so it is going to be real hard to change that. It's almost like I have to live up to that reputation even though I want to change.

Signed,
Sean, the Show-off
(Cindy in girls' version)

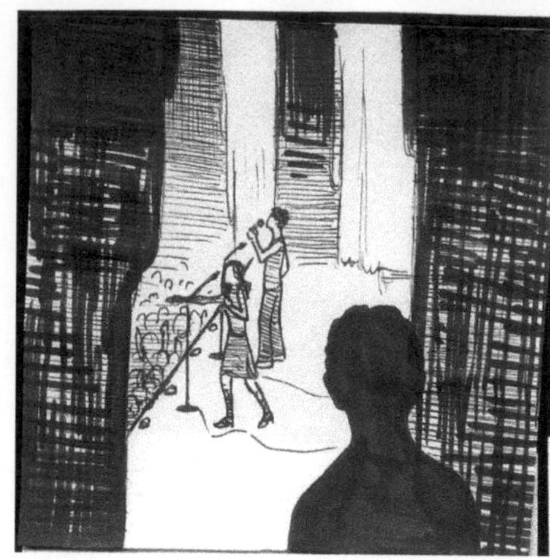

Boys' Group #3

Leo: In your letter, what your problem was—you don't have a problem!
Therapist: That's not that helpful, Leo.
Brendan: I think you should learn to say "good job" to other people.

MN: Now that was good advice.
GD: I was surprised that he spoke because he was a very shut-down child. His own self-esteem was very low.
MN: He would like someone to say "good job" to him. He's put his wish into a good suggestion for the letter-writer. In its own way, it's a generous gesture.
GD: He needs to be noticed.

Oliver: I think he should say, "Ha, ha, ha, ha. In your face!"
Therapist: You think he should do that on purpose? That's his problem and why he's writing to you. What's your real advice?

MN: You cut through his defensiveness really nicely there, in such a way that he didn't feel threatened or embarrassed.

Oliver: My advice—whenever you win, don't exaggerate. That's not hard for me because I don't usually win and I've gotten so used to losing. Next time you find yourself winning and you're "Ha-ha!," do this: either run into a tree or just sit down and concentrate really hard and get that thought out of your head. Just treat winning and losing as a daily basis of life. That's what I do.

GD: That's very sad.
MN: I agree and I'm uncomfortable with Oliver's comment about running into a tree, hurting himself. This implied the need to punish himself rather than problem-solving. It's interesting that he is sharing it. But it's very concerning.
GD: I worried a lot about Oliver turning his distress inward and developing self-destructive behaviors.

Nate: Also, when you lose, gloat really loud about losing and yell in their face. "In your face!"

Justin: First of all, here's the big thing here. You've got two possibilities. You can keep doing what you're doing or try to get away from it. It all comes down to a big root. Winning or losing. It's an attitude fact. Here's the big thing. The million-dollar question. Do you want to be a winner and a poor sport or a loser who's a good sport? (Someone exclaims, "No!") Outdoing is simple really. Think about trying to outdo something that you could never do. Have somebody tell you a story about doing something without outdoing. Remember the million dollar question!

MN: It was convoluted and idiosyncratically expressed, but there was still some good content in there.

GD: I had to distill it in order to get it.

MN: It was an interesting idea to purposely try something that you're not good at. He may not have known it, but he was picking up the bravado and the loneliness evoked by the writer. He also understood the out-of-control quality of that trait. He was coming up with something that externally could help the letter-writer stop his behaviors. The letter-writer was always so competitive, but Justin said to him: "try something that you're not good at and you won't win."

GD: Justin had worked very hard to overcome some very big challenges for himself. He was extremely hypersensitive to sounds and had to work through thresholds on a biological level just to stay in the room when the boys would laugh or talk. He had had huge obstacles that he had to master, so he was attending to this in his comment. I admired his courage in all that he had accomplished for himself.

MN: He was also, on a cognitive level and despite the convoluted quality, trying to put his thinking in order. "This is the main thing." He started with a suggestion which was pretty good, moved to a conclusion, then he went back to remember the "main thing." Despite a few left turns, the boys in this session were listening to each other. They weren't talking directly to each other, as we might have preferred, but they were using other comments made by group members in the service of formulating their own.

Jamie: First of all, forget about when you lose, you gloat. (Laughs) OK, let's get serious. And if you feel that you're about to gloat to somebody, you should just say it in your head. People might be nicer to you. And also, if you ever do lose, never mind that! If you're looking for games where you're good at, find someone who is really good so you'll have a real challenge. Bye.

MN: Despite the presentation, he's also getting it. There's some advice here that has some meaning—to work with someone who will really challenge you and make it hard.

GD: And developing competence where it should be as opposed to bravado.

MN: What nobody is touching is that the letter-writer feels really undone when he loses, as show-offs usually do. Showing off is a reaction formation. This kid feels like he's nobody and he's worthless if he doesn't win. This aspect of the letter is so hard for these vulnerable boys to respond to.

GD: Exactly. There must have been something very genuine in the voice of the letter-writer, the vulnerability that he felt, and the distress at being in this state. Justin, in his next response, I think is responding to the likeability of the boy in the letter.

Justin: I just want to quickly say, "Just do your best." At least you're not lazy, arrogant, vain.

MN: The writer is arrogant but he's also in pain that undermines the arrogance. I think Justin is empathizing with the pain.

GD: While this group was in progress, I remember that Leo was being very disruptive during this particular discussion. He was tipping his chair back, reaching and grabbing things—a lot of monkey business. He wanted the microphone, so I said . . . .

Therapist: Leo, I'm happy to let you talk if this is serious.

Leo: First I'd like to give my opinion on this little thing. I think when he wins and he starts to gloat, I think he should do what tigers do when they see a rhino charging. Run like idiots for the nearest tree.

GD: What a boy response! (Laughing) His response, however, shows the need to escape from the vulnerability that he feels.

MN: Which he has been doing the whole session. He doesn't like this topic at all.

GD: Any time we had a game in the group, Leo had to be in control of it and if he lost or his team lost, he would fall apart to the point that I had to take him out in the hallway to calm him down. This letter really spoke to him.

MN: And sadly, he couldn't deal with it! He's using escape/avoidance as a defense. "Get me out of here! This is scary and I'm in danger! My self-esteem is in danger of crashing! I have to flee!"

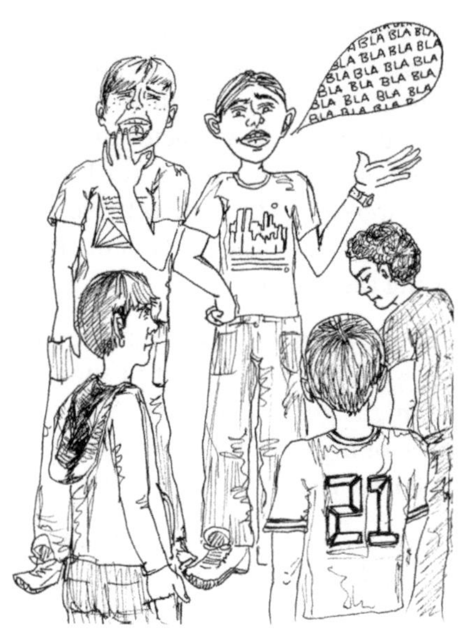

Boys' Group #1

Henry: Your problem is that you have a big ego. You need to work on that.

Therapist: You're thinking that he has a big ego. Is it really that, or something else? Is his ego small, tiny and he's trying to make it look big on purpose? Do you know what I'm saying? An inferiority complex.

MN: You picked out an aspect of the letter that could help them, and at the right time. It's a good demonstration of the quick decisions we're called on to make, particularly in group therapy where things happen sometimes too fast.

Jacob: What you could do is wait until next year, go to another school, and change your reputation. Pretend that you were never at your old school and try to change your reputation. That takes a lot of time.

GD: Jacob, in fact, did that. He was forced to change schools because he was so out-of-control. Classmates and teachers disliked him very much. At the time of this session, Jacob was just in the process of adjusting to a new school himself.

MN: Was he speaking accurately? Had he been able to get a hold of himself and improve his reputation?

GD: It was too soon to say.

Therapist: Do you have any experience with that, changing schools?

Jacob: Yes, but I liked the other school.

GD: He hated that he was thrown out of his old school.

MN: This may well be a face-saving statement; it has just a touch of sadness.

Tyrone: If you feel like people don't want to be around you because you're bragging too much, just think about how other people feel. When you feel jealous, think about the other people around listening to you. The other people might make up stories that they're better than the other person.

MN: That level of empathy was very unusual in a boy this age.

GD: Tyrone often found himself in situations where he was the underdog—out-run, last one picked, or overlooked by peers because of his extreme shyness, motor incoordination, and learning disabilities. I think he was speaking from the heart when he said, "just think how other people feel." He knows too well what it's like to be left out for the wrong reasons.

Henry: He could be lying. Think that there's always someone better than you in some things. Try to think about that. You can't be the best at everything.

MN: The group was processing its own material. Henry was responding directly to Tyrone's comment.

Therapist: That's true. Part of it is getting used to the idea that some things you're good at, and other things you're not good at. Accepting that part of yourself.

Tyrone: Like there could be someone in your school who is good at academics or sports, but not everyone can be good at everything at one time. Everyone has their own talents and specialties.

Javier: I have a competitive spirit too. I get very competitive whenever I play someone at a sport or a game. I always get really disappointed whenever I don't make it, or my team doesn't win. The main thing is just to work at it. It works. Tell yourself that you have the ability to not do this.

MN: It is delightful to hear how these boys responded to what each other were saying. Although Javier was particularly drawn to the competition issue, he was still resonating to the process, to a piece of what Tyrone had said: "not everyone can be good at everything." He may be thinking about what he's not good at.

Henry: I'm not competitive at all. I don't like it at all. There's always somebody gloating in your face.

Therapist: Would you be competitive if they weren't that way to you?
Henry: Yeah.
Therapist: They crowd you out?
Henry: Yeah.
Therapist: How can you be competitive which is natural for some of you, and allow you the opportunity to win, but at the same time not make the other guy feel terrible if he loses to you? That's an interesting question that everyone is asking here.
Javier: You have to draw the line between happy about whether you've won and bragging about winning. There's a line that can be crossed.

MN: Javier's comment was surprisingly insightful from a youngster who was so concerned with competition.
GD: Javier inspired me with his genuineness, his willingness to look at himself, and his capacity to work on improving his interpersonal skills.

Tyrone: Last year my basketball won every game that we played. The other teams got mad at us because we were winning and showing off. Towards the end of the season we started realizing how to win without showing off as much.
Therapist: That's a good way to learn how to do it.
Henry: My team never wins so I know what it's like to be the loser.

GD: This poor kid had "Loser" written all over his face. The discussion in this group session had a clear trajectory. It started with the big ego, competition.
MN: Then the boys talked about what it felt like to be on the receiving end of losing, circling back to the competition issue itself.
GD: And it finally ended with a child who was on the receiving end of losing. It was very poignant. I liked the shape of this discussion.
MN: I do, too. It had a real flow—beginning, middle, and end. I feel like the boys did their best to traverse the material.
GD: They were truly dealing with the material in this letter.

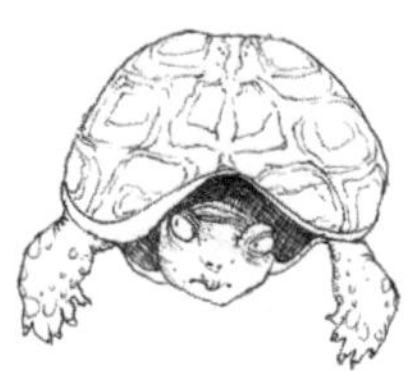

Suggested Activities

1. Videotape the group members as they create a story with their town of dioramas.
2. Encourage the children to tell something that happened that week that bothered them. Have several children describe "just the facts" of the story like a police detective. Several children act out the story. The group leader stops action to inquire what the different players might be thinking. A "thought bubble" can be drawn on a piece of paper and held over the child's head to convey the idea that we want to know what's going on inside their head. Continue the action of the story, then pause again to inquire how the actors are feeling. A heart can be drawn on a piece of paper and held over the child's head to help children focus on their feelings. These techniques can be interspersed throughout the role-play. The group leader can

assign the role of "judge" to one or more children not involved in role-playing. The judge's role is to come up with solutions to the problem that take into account what the players are thinking and feeling.

References

Greenspan, S. I. (1993). *Playground politics: The emotional development of your school-aged child.* Reading, MA: Addison-Wesley.

Heaney, C. A., & Israel, A. (2002). Social networks and social support. In K. Glanz, F. Lewis, & B. Rimer (Eds.), *Health behavior and health education: Theory, research and practice* (3rd ed., pp. 185–209). San Francisco: Jossey-Bass.

CHAPTER 6
To Be or Who to Be
The Question for Parents and the Budding Adolescent

As we continue to explore the theme of how identity develops, the following letter addresses the changes that a pre-adolescent child experiences during this process. Some children are embarrassed by or ashamed of these changes. Other children take on a new appearance, identifying with a pop culture or sub-group to announce to the world who they are, or whom they now believe themselves to be (Sullivan, 1953; Greenspan, 2002). The identification with a particular group can be met with both approval and disapproval by parents and peers. In this particular letter, the child's parents have a version of what they want the child to look and act like that differs from the child's. The group sessions that follow demonstrate both normative identity-formation concerns as well as those particular to youngsters experiencing the interaction of regulatory disorders and intrapsychic factors.

Dear Kids' Club,

I am thirteen years old and am a total geek. I am overweight and dumpy looking and as I have entered adolescence, I have started getting zits. I am really embarrassed by the changes in my body. I'm sure you know what I am talking about. My parents always say, "Oh, look how you're growing!"

So here is the real problem. My parents want me to dress in really retarded-looking clothes. No one at my school wears these things. When I wear what I like, my parents really disapprove and give me a hard time. I actually stashed some good clothes in my locker at school and change secretly so they don't know. I can't go through life being ashamed, not just of my weight problem, but of the geeky clothes they make me wear. Even when I wear the clothes that I like so I can fit in better with the other kids, I feel like it's all a big joke. It's not really me because I have to hide it from my parents who want me to be someone else.

Recently I have started hanging out with a cool crowd. They are into Goth—wear black all the time, do their hair cool, and talk a lot about death and feeling depressed. Actually, I am really like that—depressed, so I don't have to make up those thoughts when we talk about who feels the dumpiest inside. I really like hanging out with them. My parents found out about the Goth crowd, even though I tried hard to hide it from them. They are all worked up about it, saying I am going to ruin myself for good. These kids understand me. I feel like I finally fit in somewhere.

What would you do if you were in my shoes?

Signed,
George, the Geek, now transformed Goth
Laura (Girls' version)

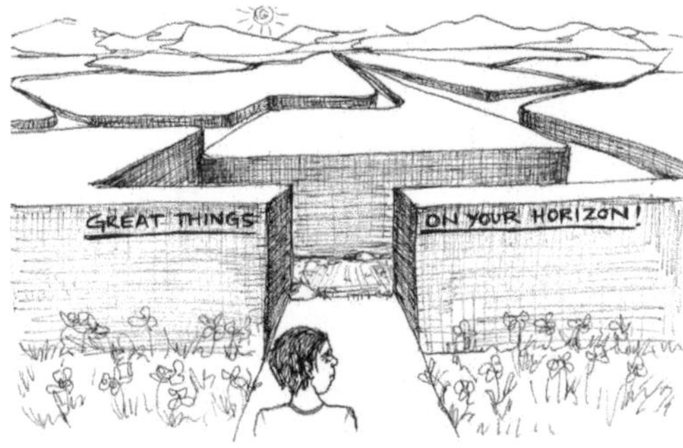

GD: I didn't know which parts of the letter they would focus on. There are a number of things that this letter could elicit. What comes to mind are the self-image issues, the changes in the body, and the clothes struggle. There is also the part about not living up to their parents' expectations, parents not understanding them, or the pull to be in a crowd that fits them even though it's so discrepant from their parents' wishes. I tried to put different layers in the letter to see to what each group might resonate.

Girls' Group #3

Alexis: I think what you should do is wear what you want to wear. Just tell your mom and dad how you feel that you don't fit in wearing the clothes they want you to wear. Sometimes, though, you have to compromise. Once I really wanted to wear a fancy dress to school. I wanted to show the kids this special dress I was going to wear to my birthday party. My mom refused me. I threw a big fit but later we agreed on something I could wear that wouldn't be so fancy. Besides that though, you should wear what you want. You want to be true to yourself.

MN: The group began by paying attention to appearance being the primary defining aspect of identity. By 13, kids should be picking out their clothes. It's part of self-expression, and a way of trying-on different "identities" in an age-appropriate way. I think that parental limits should be confined to clothing that is too provocative or obviously outrageous, like very revealing clothing for girls. Goth dress is, though, rather disturbing to most parents, and suggests identification with a particular type of youngster who cultivates alienation. Goth-affiliation is indeed worrisome to therapists as well as parents.

GD: In Alexis's case, her focus on appearance coincided with her own need to be admired for her looks. She was going in the right direction when she says, "you want to be true to yourself." Finding her real self and allowing others to see this was very challenging for her.

Therapist: That's a very good suggestion, Alexis. Does anybody have anything to say about the girl identifying with the Goth crowd and what she should do about that?

Deborah: I say that if she really likes the Goth kids, she should see them. It seems that she is comfortable talking with them about how she feels. The only problem is that the kids who aren't Goth will not hang out with her if she only sees them, so maybe she could hang out half the time with the Goth kids and the other half with the regular kids. That way her parents will approve of some of her friends.

MN: Deborah picked up on Alexis's comment about compromise.

GD: I was startled that Deborah was able to say this. She could be described as an outlier, with no friends. She had no peer group of her own, so I was surprised that she was able to make that observation.

MN: These girls seem to have understood the youngster in the letter.

Therapist: That's a great way for her to meet her own needs and satisfy her parents' wishes as well. What about her feeling depressed? We haven't helped her with that problem.

Gillian: I can say something about that because I am depressed inside. I know how that feels.

Therapist: Can you say more?

Gillian: I really hate the way my face looks and other things, too. (Gillian was the youngster with cerebral palsy.) I look at my face and I wish it was different. It's not easy for me to say this.

Therapist: That took a lot of courage to say that today to this group. Even though this letter is about Laura who feels this way, we have a girl right here in this group who feels depressed about how she looks. Let's help her out because that will also make Laura feel good that she helped another girl with what she said. What can we say right now to Gillian to help her?

GD: Gillian made herself available on a much deeper level than she normally would do, revealing something very important to the group. I wanted to support her self-disclosure and encourage the group to do so as well.

MN: You very nicely placed yourself on the therapeutic periphery of the group. By that I mean that you posed a problem for the group to consider, that was based on the group's own material, asked the group to think about it, and then backed up. The fact that you did this demonstrates a clinical decision that therapists must make regarding how central or peripheral they should make themselves in the course of any group session. The position we take should always be fluid.

Ashley: Gillian, none of us can change our faces and how they look, but we can work on other things about ourselves, like improving things we do by practicing. I did that with gymnastics and I ended up becoming really good at it. When I felt low about myself in other ways, I just said to myself, "See, you are good at something. The rest doesn't matter so much."

MN: How lovely and empathic Ashley was able to be. This whole section of the group's process was so poignantly productive. They were being vulnerable in front of each other; they were resonating to the letter; and they were being thoughtful on a group level as well. You can see that they needed less intervention from you. That is something we want in a good group. You were saying much less here because you don't need to. On one level, you were demonstrating one therapeutic goal: we are in the paradoxical professional position of working with each patient so that we can eventually become obsolete!

GD: Just the fact that a girl stepped forward in the way she did in this group, to expose her innermost self, was impressive and courageous. My decision was to drop the letter and attend to that girl's need.

MN: You clearly didn't need the letter anymore.

Therapist: What we're talking about is building up things we can change about ourselves. It's called "self-improvement." Gillian, I'm thinking right now about how you like to play basketball. Is that something that helps you to feel better about yourself?

Gillian: Yes, sometimes.

Therapist: It seems that it doesn't change how you feel about your face though. You are really sad about that, and we should talk more about this, as you feel ready to share with the girls here.

GD: It seemed the right time for me to interject a focus for the group. I remember Gillian turning to me and whispering that she wanted individual treatment time with me. That was the setting where she could talk more about these feelings.

MN: She did some here in the group and went as far as she could at the time. She observed herself and her feelings and knew this. She also knew that she needed more time to talk about it and to do so more privately. She was essentially meeting her own needs-assessment and following through!

GD: This also raised the therapeutic issue of when to segue from group to individual treatment and how to interweave the two. What are the boundaries and limits of each modality of treatment? How do you triage them so both modalities are used at the right time?

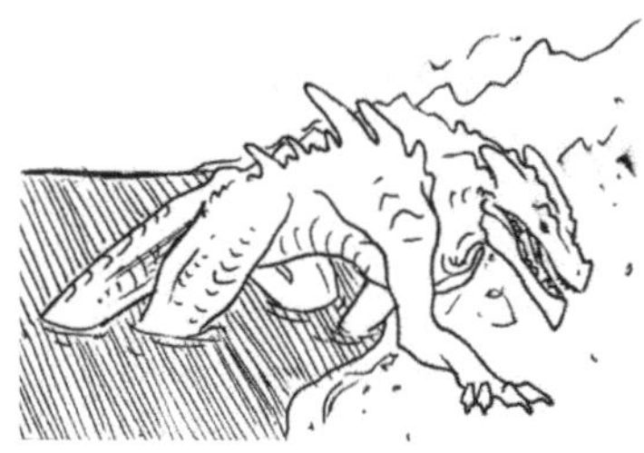

Girls' Group #5

Nadia: If your parents want you to wear retarded clothes and you don't really feel like it, say, "Mom, it's not really cool to wear retarded clothes. People make fun of me." Boys might not like you. If your mom says you have to, say it's not fair.

GD: It was a big accomplishment for Nadia to have said this because she was very shy and withdrawn. If she were to stand up to her own mother, it would have been a major achievement.

Brooke: My name is Brooke.

MN: Brooke broke the process by her self-involved comment. There was no reason for her to introduce herself to girls she'd been with for a long time. However, after this interruption, she did get herself back into the group.

Brooke: Maybe your mom doesn't really doesn't understand that you don't like those clothes. Say to her, "Mom, I don't really like those clothes that much. Maybe we could go shopping for some new clothes." Tell her, "I really want new clothes. Everyone makes fun of me and I look like a dork." And tell her thanks for buying you new clothes.

Melissa: I think what you should do and it really works for me is when my mom wants to buy me clothes that I don't feel like wearing, say, "You can waste your money, but I'm not going to wear these clothes." She says, "Fine, you can pick out clothes but you're going to wear two pairs of clothes that I buy." That's how we work it.

MN: I don't know whether to call this a power struggle or a negotiation. It was really both. Melissa described a dynamic between her and her mother that they would fall into. She had the tone of someone who enjoyed creating the struggle. Perhaps Melissa perceived the power struggles as a necessary part of her relationship with her mother, or, better put: Melissa believed that she required a power struggle with her mother because without it they wouldn't have a relationship. The issue of power struggle and standoff versus negotiation had entered the group conversation.

GD: Melissa and her mother locked horns over many kinds of struggles. I had a hard time making inroads trying to change how they interacted with one another. In a way, Melissa's mother was teaching Melissa how to have a power struggle rather than how to negotiate.

Therapist: You negotiate. None of us has talked to her about her problem of feeling depressed inside. Does anybody want to share anything about that? Anything that you've done when you feel sad or not so good about yourself?

Nadia: Once my mom told me to wear these clothes and I didn't feel like it. Like last night we had dress-up day at school, and I wanted to wear this red dress. She said, "No, it's going to be all muddy." And I said, "Come on, please." She said no and I was really depressed because I really wanted to wear it.

GD: She was avoiding the real issue. She got stuck on what this girl was wearing rather than what she was feeling inside.

MN: Yes. The clothes were a symbol. Nadia described a dynamic between her and her mother, and then told us about her internalized reaction to their interaction. There was a relational conflict; she would yield, and then have feelings about it, most likely anger because she reported that she then became depressed. We are seeing both the relational and the internalized, dynamic aspects at work in this youngster's comment.

Therapist: You know it sounds like everyone is still thinking about the clothes problem and it makes me wonder if everyone thinks that Laura is depressed because she can't get her parents to let her wear clothes that she likes. Is that why you think she's depressed?

Brittany: Well, today when me and my mom were yelling at each other, and my mom said that only God was her friend and that my Dad and I were the only ones who didn't care about her. That made me really depressed inside when I got to school, but I told her that my Dad and I do care about her a whole lot and we do worry about her too. And she said, "That's OK" or "I forgive you."

MN: If that was true, then she was privy to what she shouldn't have been privy to. She had accepted the job of taking care of her mother. Youngsters can only fail at such a job because children are never equipped to be the parent of a parent. This almost inevitably leads to feelings of helplessness and ineffectiveness that can affect one's identity for years to come.

GD: I also worked with Brittany individually. Her mother was very fragile and had borderline traits. Whatever her child felt inevitably got transformed into her own problem. It was very difficult for me to figure out whose feelings were whose. Her mother frequently fell apart and Brittany did her best to try to take care of her. What was even sadder was that Brittany had originally come from a family in which she was abused physically and sexually.

MN: The nature of Brittany's relationship with her mother, and she was telling the group about it, made me wonder for whom she was adopted and for what purpose. This particular letter was leading the youngsters to evoke people outside the group. They were bringing their parents into the room, and they shifted away from the focus on clothes.

GD: That was one of the things I wanted to do: bring in the social and emotional layers each child experiences. I'm glad the girls were able to do this and that they could disclose their relationships to their parents, at least within this particular group session.

Therapist: Anybody else? We hope this is helpful. Bye, Laura.

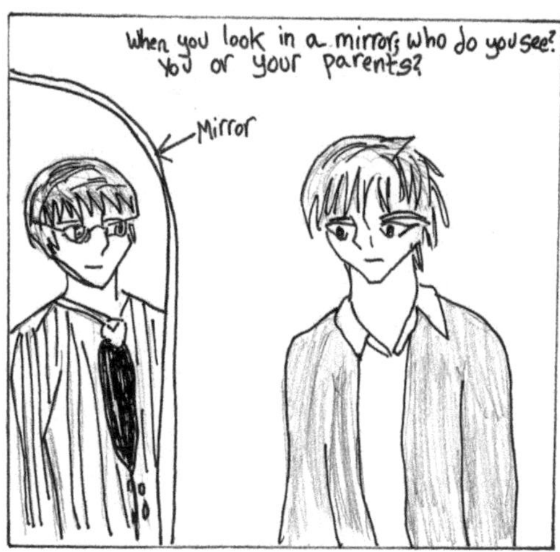
When you look in a mirror, who do you see? You or your parents?
Mirror

Boys' Group #2

Kevin: My personal motto is, what they don't know can't hurt them.
Therapist: Parents?

Kevin: Yep. What the parents don't know can't hurt them.

Therapist: So what's your advice?

Kevin: If you really want to join the club, tell your parents you really insist on it and you can't have any other way. Try to explain to them and if they refuse, well, you might have to do it anyway because if it is a place you really fit in, then it's good for you.

Therapist: I just wanted to mention something, Kevin. When I was reading the letter, Kevin, you said, "Join the club!" Can you explain a little bit about that?

GD: He said, "Join the club!" about mid-way into my reading of the letter.

MN: This is a good example of how even a simple three-word sentence can have multiple meanings as well as be a metaphor. Kevin's comment was actually rather elegant as an act of communication: "Join the club!" In providing guidance to help the letter-writer fit in with the Goth crowd, Kevin was also expressing how alien he could feel in general. His "club" was that of all his own peers, from whom he felt alienated. He conveyed his own loneliness. A great example of layered communication.

Kevin: Well, I was depressed. Yeah. Depressed a lot. Almost everyone is. Especially me after a string of bad luck. I almost got used to saying curse words like 50 times a day.

Manuel: I say curse words all the time too but in my head.

GD: Kevin was articulating the complexities of his own depression and how it had led to anger turned inward. Somehow his self-disclosure helped Manuel to speak about his own internal world. Normally Manuel would not say anything during an entire group, being shut-down, uncommunicative, and scowling at the other kids. At last he had opened up to tell them that he engaged in negative self-talk, and that anger and frustration lived in his head.

MN: Kevin's had been speaking for the group. He first voiced his alienation from the interpersonal world around him. Then he labeled his depression and even took it further and let us know about his underlying anger. Kevin was obviously **not** alone with his anger. Manuel wanted Kevin to know this, even as Manuel spoke about himself. The communication of one group member with another was evident in the timing of the comments.

GD: Nicely articulated too.

Julian: Here's an idea (said in carnival barker-like voice). Just wait a while. Wait until your parents forget.

Therapist: There's nothing like a stalling tactic!

Julian: Hang out with the Goth club again. By the way, throw out the geeky clothes and claim that the dog ate them.

MN: This statement was funny, but it presented a difficulty for a group therapist. Julian was actually heading somewhere very serious at this moment. The trick for the therapist would be to quietly appreciate the absurd, although age-appropriate, humor in this tactic, while continuing to listen seriously.

GD: I chose to wait and see where his use of humor might go.

Julian: That also works sometimes. I haven't tried it but it probably will work.

MN: He started to speak, subtly, of his hopelessness.

GD: Julian often felt demoralized that nothing worked for him. He was so overwhelmed by his lack of interpersonal effectiveness and coping abilities that he usually did nothing or something outrageously inappropriate.

Therapist: I want to ask you if anyone has found something that helps you when you feel down and depressed.

Julian: Here's a bit of advice that is something that you shouldn't do. For example, ummm . . . .

MN: A therapist needs to note that pause: "ummm."

GD: By the group waiting and honoring his anxiety, they gave him the space to speak more.

Julian: I used to hurt myself when I was depressed. What do you know? I was depressed all the time. Sigh. I wasn't into pain, but what the heck!

GD: There it was! His self-revelation was poignant. I hoped that in speaking of his depression to the group, he would feel our support and thus, lessen his internal pain. He was a head-banger and sometimes did it during group when he was upset.

Therapist: So what's your advice?

Julian: Don't beat yourself up! Trust me on this one.

Therapist: You used to hurt yourself. How did you stop that habit because some kids do that when they don't like themselves or are so mad at themselves?

Julian: I didn't. I just stopped being depressed all the time. OK. You're asking me about this is making me depressed.

GD: Julian had had enough. He had reached his tolerance level for sharing these intense feelings.

MN: We might also see his comment in a process way: he was saying he could take no more and wanted the group to know it.

GD: This was one of the benefits of group psychotherapy—when one cannot tolerate the intensity of affect, it was sometimes easier to retreat and allow another person to step forward. But when that didn't happen, it could lead to more distress for a group member which was what happened next in this sequence.

Therapist: OK. He's banging his head here (Julian actually was doing it!).

Manuel: I keep it in my head. I do nothing. Don't bottle it up.

GD: I was stunned that Manuel said this because he was almost always quiet in group. He was saying that he kept it in his head and held it inside, yet his advice was "Don't bottle it up."

MN: Despite Julian's comment, the topic was so strong that the group couldn't stop its process. Manuel was saying what he would do—I keep it in my head and bottle it up. He seemed aware that this was problematic for him. Interestingly, he also had the solution but didn't use it. I find Manuel plaintive because he was the same youngster who was empathically responding to Kevin just a few minutes ago.

Julian: Don't bottle it up! It makes you go insane! Trust me! Argh!

Therapist: You're acting silly about it, but if a person does feel sad inside, you're not cuckoo. Everyone in this room has had these feelings.

Kevin: I'm not crazy. Just mentally retarded.

GD: He was a brilliant child with Asperger's. I think that he doubted his intelligence because people were always correcting him or telling him to stop doing something inappropriate.

MN: So he was talking about his misfit status, just as he was earlier: "Join the club."

Aidan: Quiet! Let's be serious! If you're feeling upset and you want to join their club.

GD and MN: (almost simultaneously) Right on target!

Aidan: Maybe your parents have some good ideas and use their background knowledge from what they know. You may need to ask your parents, if you can get the time to know them enough, that you can make your own decision about who you're going to be friends with. You can also tell them, "I don't have many friends and I'm trying to fit in. Right now, it feels like you're bugging me about it. Now I don't have many friends again. And I don't feel good about these clothes because they're not what's cool. Everybody except me thinks I'm strange and ugly and not cool." You can tell them that you have to switch clothes to fit in. "You're making me wear these clothes!"

Therapist: That's excellent advice, Aidan.

MN: It sounds like he had good, available parents whom he thought could be helpful to him. His description of them suggests that he trusted them.

GD: His mother spent a lot of time processing things with Aidan, helping him understand himself and his behavior. He had enormous problems over the years with impulse control and fitting in. He had struggled with being liked.

Julian: Also, I was going to say that you have to make sure. Tell them that, well, how do I say this?

MN: Again, a group member offered a pregnant pause. Something that was hard for him to say was coming. Julian was the boy who had earlier said that he had reached a saturation point with the discussion. At this moment, he was able to re-enter it.

Julian: Tell them people staring at you makes you feel depressed and dumpy, etc. etc.

MN: He was articulating the details of the social process. He was offering a follow-up comment. The boys were working together as a group quite well. Their process was responsive, reciprocal, on-target, and really not evasive.

Kevin: OK. Also tell your parents that you know they feel that they know what's best for you, but you need to lay down a few rules for them, too. They can't control your life too. You also need to make some rules and put some rules down for them. They're giving you too many orders. Also, sometimes, not respecting their wishes may come about in a positive result because they realize that you're not following their rules. It only makes matters worse. Stop whatever it is—wearing those geeky clothes, or joining the Goth group.

MN: I don't follow Kevin's meaning completely, but the oppositional quality of the statement is clear. I assume that this was age-appropriate bravado that also may have been serving a defensive function.

Therapist: You have a lot of different advice here. Not telling your parents and doing it anyhow, or maybe listening to your parents, or being honest.

Aidan: I said you should try to compromise with them. I didn't say you shouldn't listen to your parents. Perhaps they would let you get to know these people (the Goths) to see if they really are people that could be your friends. Because they (the parents) could be right or they could be wrong.

MN: Aidan was responding to Kevin's oppositional qualities and by being more reasonable, compromising, and thoughtful. He was considering both the child and parent's viewpoints. This required empathy.

GD: I was surprised that Aidan could come up with something this insightful and balanced and not get into the thick of it with Kevin, because that was usually what would happen in group—the two of them going after one another. He stayed on-topic and stayed focused.

Therapist: Right. Your point is to figure out how to negotiate with your parents. The other important thing you said, Aidan, is that you don't want to lie to your parents because it will come back and bite you in the end. The other point that Kevin was making is that kids have opinions. Parents should hear what those opinions are.

Kevin: Lay down some rules for them.

Therapist: Compromise is important as part of that process.

Aidan: Sometimes that can be helpful. If you lay down rules for them, they could become upset that you are taking over. You could say, "I feel like this is happening and we should have this happen instead." It's too demanding to lay down rules for your parents. You should ask them to take down a few rules and make the rules more reasonable and to give you more space.

GD: I think that this group demonstrated an excellent process. The boys expressed heart-wrenching feelings, offered support in a non-judgmental way to one another, and tolerated the distress of the feelings that got stirred up in the group. Then they came full-circle to offer helpful strategies not only to the letter-writer but also to one another. I was impressed by their work.

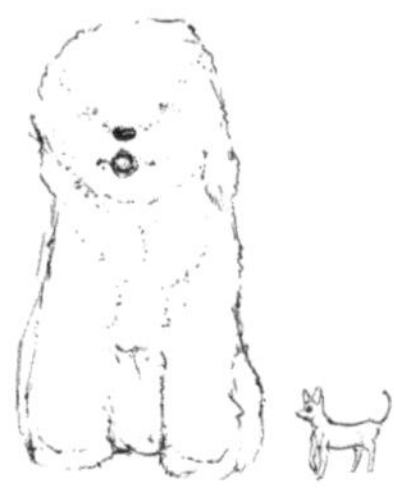

Suggested Activities

1. Ask each child to list five adjectives that describe how they see themselves, how their friends see them, and how their parents see them. Prompt them with the following questions:
   a. Which ones are the real you?
   b. What makes you feel happiest about yourself?

c. Are there any changes that you want to make in yourself?

A variation of this activity is to have each child write their name on a piece of paper, then pass the paper to the child to their right. That child writes down an adjective about the child whose paper it is. The paper continues to circulate around the table until it returns to its owner. The group then discusses what was elicited.

2. Draw a picture of yourself and how you wish you could be.
3. Bring pictures to the group next week of yourself at different ages to share.

References

Greenspan, S. I. (2002). *The secure child*. Cambridge, MA: Perseus Books.
Sullivan, H. S. (1953). *The interpersonal theory of psychiatry*. New York: W.W. Norton.

CHAPTER 7
An Unfocused Lens
The ADHD Child's Perspective

This next letter tries to capture the experience of children with ADHD who constantly struggles with time management and organization. Their distractibility and problems processing information, particularly verbal directions, is their nemesis. They always feel rushed with no time to relax and to refuel an already overburdened nervous system. Their daily experience of life is of their parents and teachers repeatedly nagging them to get to places on time, to get dressed in the morning, to keep their room organized, and to finish their homework. It is an endless list of demands that swims in their already flooded head. It is too much for them to process at once and to execute. Their impulses to touch and do things that pop into their head in the moment are criticized by everyone (Brown, 2005; Levine, 2003; Sommers-Flanagan & Sommers-Flanagan, 2002).

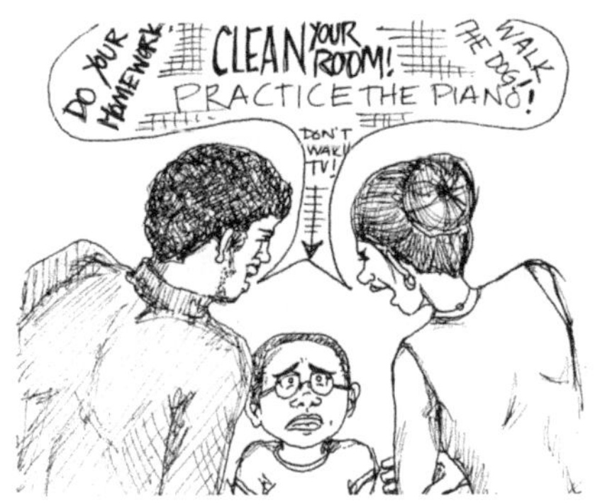

Dear Kids' Club,

I have ADHD—attention deficit disorder with hyperactivity! When I say, hyperactive, I mean hyperactive. I am always on the go—an active sort of kid. I don't mind being so active, but what bothers me about having ADHD is that I cannot get anything done on time. My day starts out with my mom yelling at me to "Get out of bed! Get dressed, already! You're going to miss the bus again!" When I'm at school, I seem to miss things that the teacher says and then I come home missing half the homework assignments. I just tell my mom that I don't have to worry about science or math, even though they probably had an assignment. My mom yells at me that I have to start getting things straight. She says, "Just write it down when the teacher tells you what the homework is!" She doesn't know that I sometimes don't hear it, or I forget to write it down from the chalk board. When I start on the homework, I can't sit still. I feel like jumping out of my skin. I need to move, especially after sitting all day at school. I keep begging my mom for a break, and she just says, "You have wasted 45 minutes complaining!" Then on weekends, my parents hassle me about the mess in my bedroom. What kid my age has a nasty neat bedroom! My mom starts yelling, "Pick up your dirty laundry. What am I, your maid?" I have no time to chill out. I feel like a slave to work. Plus my mom is one big fat yelling mama. I can't stand my life. I think the problem is that my ADHD makes me be this way. Is there anything a person like me can do to make it better? I feel trapped in my body, in my house, in a completely overwhelming life.

Signed,
Adam, Mr. ADHD
(Amy in girl's version)

Girls' Group #2

Chelsea: Before you do your homework, you should try to relax or by super glue.

MN: Was she in earnest or was that her sense of humor?
GD: I think it was her sense of humor. This was how I responded.

Therapist: Super Glue! What does that have to do with it?
Chelsea: Sit on the super glue.
Maya: I think that the problem is that you are really active and you should run around outside first before you do your homework.
Therapist: That's a good idea. Some of you here might try that.

MN: Were there kids in this group who did have ADHD?
GD: Yes. Chelsea had ADHD and so did Briana. Danielle had ADD with a hyperfocus problem.
MN: So Chelsea could make an empathic connection. When she made the comment about the Super Glue, she may have been aware that the letter-writer couldn't control herself and needed some external support. So the Super Glue was a metaphor for the out-of-control experience.
GD: I was surprised that she had the capacity to make that connection. We really need to remember how much children use metaphors. They're easy to miss because there's so much going on at once in any group session.

Briana: I think that the best idea would be to do your homework after relaxing for a little while, then get up and go play for as long as you can because that will get all your jitters out of you. You could always go outside and play after a little while. Then when you come back inside, you're relaxed and ready to work.

GD: Her language reflects an ADHD kind of mind. She understood the need for variety.

MN: She's learned about the need for tension reduction and then alternating between honing in on what you need to do, really concentrating, and then taking a break. She told the group that she understood some coping strategies and that she had some realistic sense of herself as a person with ADHD. I also hear a degree of self-acceptance.

GD: It's a nice example of how children, and not only children with ADHD, need repeated breaks, something that not all parents understand. However, a normal nervous system doesn't have the kind of urgent cycling that the child with ADHD has in terms of activity level.

MN: So far in this session, these youngsters have focused on the personal experience of a child who had ADHD. They hadn't yet gotten to the description of the mother who didn't understand.

GD: I was curious if they could look at this issue and discuss it, because that certainly was the experience of several of these children. Actually, Maya, the child who spoke next, was able to bring her mother into the discussion.

Maya: Maybe you could make a deal with your mom that if you first do part of your homework, you could go outside for 20 minutes. Then when you come back in, do the rest of your homework.

Therapist: That's called negotiating.

Danielle: I have ADD that is a little bit like this, and sometimes I can't concentrate.

Therapist: What do you do about it, Danielle?

Danielle: My advice is to try to talk to your mom and try to at least use a fidget which will help you with homework and classwork. Ask your mom or dad if you can have a bracelet that you can pull at. When you pull at the bracelet it helps to concentrate on your work.

MN: She was offering something important, but she required defensive distantiation in order to do it. She's gone from first to second person in this comment. I think this is an excellent example of a healthy use of defense. Her distantiation permits her to continue thinking about and talking about herself.

Therapist: That's very brave of you to tell Amy that you also have a problem like hers. It's not easy to bring that up in a group.

GD: Danielle was one of those youngsters who constantly buried herself in comic books or other books. I would need to ask her quietly to put her book aside and say to her that she was in a group right now and how much we wanted her to participate with us. For her to share something personal was quite significant.

MN: This segment between you and Danielle was rather nice because what you were doing was validating her, and that's what the letter-writer was saying was missing in her own life.

GD: This is the kind of parallel process that we often see in groups. Danielle's parents would like her to snap out of her issues, just as I worked with her to "snap out of" her comic book. Her parents were weary of her ongoing needs. They frequently asked me, "Is she getting anything out of the group? Won't she be better soon?"

MN: I think that we frequently overlook the fact that youngsters with these kinds of problems are very wearing on parents. Parents aren't monsters. They are worn down and need our empathy too. Often parents don't understand that ADHD is a condition their children have. It isn't a simple symptom that just abates. So the mother in the letter may not be truly unempathic in an ongoing way, but exhausted by having a youngster with ADHD. We as therapists need to remember that too.

GD: In putting that letter together, I wanted to capture what I commonly hear from parents concerning what it's like—having to drag their child out of bed every morning and constantly having to be vigilant and remind them to do things. It's very taxing for anyone to sustain that degree of oversight.

MN: All day long—including the frequent struggles over eating breakfast and dinner, because the medication often diminishes appetite. Then there are often difficulties and stubbornness about the bedtime ritual, going to bed, and actually getting to sleep. Then the whole thing starts over the next day. I'd be exhausted too!

GD: It's wearing for both parent and child to have this dynamic day in, day out.

MN: Just as the child needs empathy, so do the parents. Sometimes I think we forget that.

Briana: Here's some relaxation. You can get up and put your hands together and push on them five times really hard. You can stamp your feet on the ground and if you really want to get active, have your mom buy you a punching bag. Put it in your basement. Whenever you're really jittery go downstairs and pretend the punching bag is your little annoying brother. Punch it as hard as you can until you're all pooped. Then go back upstairs and you'll be really tired and you'll be able to work quietly.

MN: She gave a recipe and some nice advice ... except for that poor little brother, even he was annoying.

Therapist: Amy, in this group there are a lot of girls who know about this restlessness problem.

Chelsea: If you take a few minutes to do your homework, then you will have a few hours to run outside.

MN: That was a distortion because homework takes more than a few minutes. These girls were old enough to have a lot of homework. This was almost like the defense of magical thinking, to avoid what it feels like to have something as difficult as it is to live with ADHD. The child doesn't like it anymore than the parents do.

GD: Chelsea was this way about almost everything in her life. If you bought her the latest style in running shoes, she'd automatically be a superstar. There's not much work needed for that. Her mom had to harangue her regularly to practice her piano. Chelsea's idea was that if she sat down for two minutes, then she would magically know the piece. She could become an expert musician with no effort. That's how she was with everything: homework, skills that she was learning, and sports. It was a cavalier process for her.

MN: Was that attributable entirely to her ADHD, or was there also an intrapsychic element? Did she, underneath the cavalier presentation, believe that she was not good enough, that she couldn't achieve, that there was something wrong with her, that she couldn't measure up? Did she harbor the idea that she was pervasively a failure as a person? Her psychodynamics and condition (ADHD) interact with each other.

GD: I think so. It's an important point: children like Chelsea internalize an inadequate self. Many children with ADHD do.

Therapist: Does anyone have a suggestion about how to remember what the homework assignment was?

Chelsea: Same with me. (Four children raise hands)

Therapist: Four girls here are raising their hands. I was wondering if anyone has suggestions for what to do.

Danielle: Try to write down on a piece of paper the homework you're supposed to do and put it in your back pack. Then when you see it, you can get right to work. Usually at my old school, I forgot the assignments. Now I bring the paper home and know what I am supposed to do. If I have a bad assignment to do, something really hard, I write down at least a few things I need to do to get it done. My advice is if you finish it, put a happy face or a star on your paper.

MN: I like her strategy of engaging in positive self-talk: rewarding herself with that happy face.

Maya: I have 2 things. If you have a best friend you can trust, you can talk with her about it. Or you can call up a friend and ask. Write it down in a notebook or tape it in your notebook.

GD: It was so sweet that she brought a friend into the discussion.

MN: This is the first time that a child had brought in another person, instead of Super Glue™, as auxiliary support.

GD: Maya was the child who moved here and lost all her friends. You could just feel her yearning for connection in many of the things she said. But she was also resourceful, a big strength for her.

Annie: You can make a special thing with your teacher like a check list. Make sure you write it down.

MN: There was a shift in the group process away from each girl sharing with the other group members her own internal experiences, to seeking the assistance of useful outsiders like teachers. The group had sought and had found additional kinds of support that was available.

GD: What was so nice was that this wasn't from my modeling or offering support in the way I was interacting with them. It came from them. They were learning where to look for outside help.

MN: I think it began with your affirming comment to Danielle. It took the kids a little while to get to it, but they experienced it with you first, on a level that they may not have been aware of. They experienced your comments as helpful; then they were able to think about other people, including parents, and how they might be helpful.

GD: It was a nice parallel process.

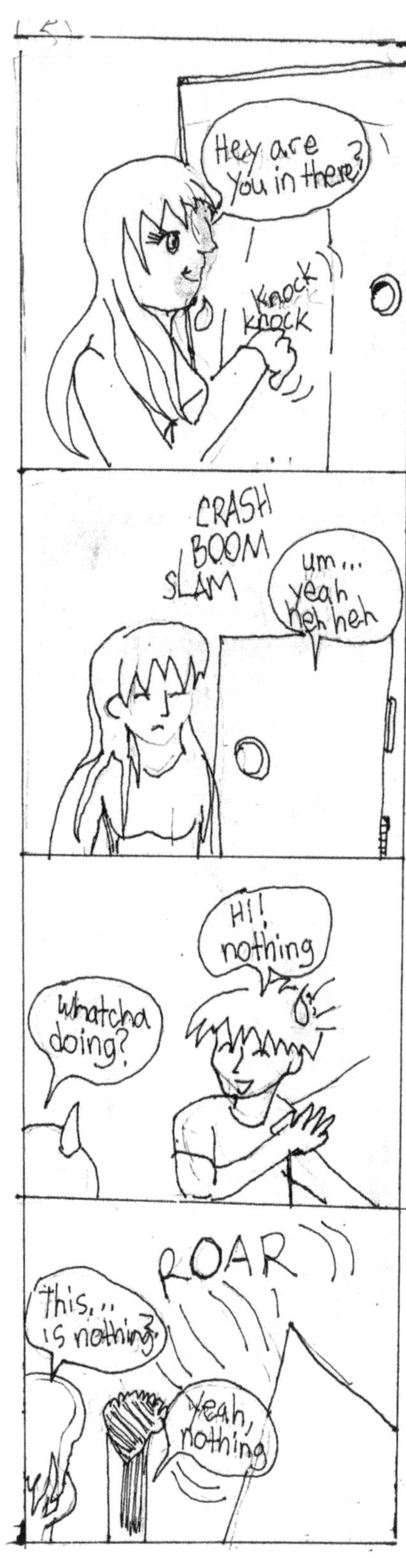
Hey are you in there?
knock knock
CRASH
BOOM
SLAM
um... yeah heh heh
Whatcha doing?
Hi! nothing
ROAR
this... is nothing?
Yeah, nothing

Girls' Group #3

Kendra: You really need an agenda book. It has all your subjects listed like Spanish, Science, and stuff like that, and you write down the homework when they say it. My teacher signs the agenda book.

Deborah: First of all, talk to your mother and explain to her about your problem. Say you want help and she can arrange to have someone work with you on your homework. Like how to stay on the topic.

MN: This group immediately sought a collaboration between self and others in trying to find helpful accommodations to the problems of a child with ADHD.

Deborah: Talk to the teacher and she can give you some post-it notes to write down the assignments. Then you can copy it down later. Also, you can confirm with a friend to see if you have any homework.

GD: That was really nice, well-articulated, and helpful advice.

MN: It was sophisticated in its way because it pulled together helpful adults (teachers), oneself, and helpful peers. Did Deborah have ADD?

GD: Yes. She also had some attributes of a child with Asperger's syndrome. She became immersed in thoughts in her head and could easily go off-topic. This comment was especially nice because Deborah was a loner and didn't use people for support. She frequently talked by writing things on paper. I was so pleased that she participated in this discussion, and in a helpful, connected way.

Therapist: There are some girls here who have ADD, having trouble paying attention. And some girls have ADHD where you are active.

Gillian: If you're hyper and you're jumping up and down and walking around, you can do exercises before you go to school, after school, and in the night. Do it before you do your homework. That helps me. I get very hyper and don't know why. Talk to your mom and say, "I'm sorry. I love you. I'm just hyper today."

MN: She was sensitive to the dynamic between parent and the child and wanted to be understood. Her perception was that the parent didn't understand that she, Gillian, couldn't help it. It was not a rejection of the mother or defiant behavior. It just was her condition and all she wanted was for her mother to be aware of that and to understand that Gillian was not intentionally trying to be difficult.

GD: It was interesting that in my ongoing work with Gillian, she became hyperactive and did impulsive things. She also had bursts of anger, when she threw things and cursed, and attacked her mother verbally. Her mother took these tension-reduction outbursts as an intentional "assault" from Gillian. I worked with them both to help them understand each other's perspective as well as understand what Gillian's anger meant. An anger outburst directed at them was actually an outbreak of frustration. It's a hard lesson for many parents because the frustration outbursts do indeed look angry and are dramatic and do require quick intervention.

MN: It wasn't a defiance of the mother for the sake of saying "I don't love you or I hate you!" She was in the grip of something she couldn't control. It was her brain, her wiring. The family dynamic would of course become much more complicated when the parent–child relationship was already troubled.

Gillian: Tell her you want to do your homework and don't want to worry about it. Sometimes I can't do my homework. Tell your mom to write a note to the teacher that you didn't have time, like you were sick or sad about something. Tell your mom and dad and family how much you love them.

GD: She needed a lot of assurance.
MN: Her perception was that her family did too.

Therapist: Great ideas. What I really like is how all of you in this group today are sharing things about yourself.
Kendra: You can tell your teachers that everyday you should get a notebook and write down the homework every single day. Also, they can sign it so that your dad and mom know you can get better grades. I also want to know what kind of grades you're getting because you have ADD.

MN: In speaking to the letter-writer, Kendra took on a parental role.
GD: Underneath, she was speaking of self-judgment and her belief that there was something inherently wrong with her. Kendra was adopted and her parents would never totally accept her for who she was. In one way or another, for them, she never quite measured up.
MN: It seemed, from her taking the parent role in her comment to the letter-writer that she had internalized the sense of being damaged.

Ashley: Every day at school the teacher writes down the homework on the board and we have to copy it down. Then everybody has to copy it down and someone comes around and checks on you. Sometimes a kid doesn't copy it down, and my teacher gets really mad and she comes around and checks everybody. That's how it works.

MN: She was reporting an empathic failure on her teacher's part. I wonder if that was because in ADHD there is sometimes a type of learning disability involving not being able to take what's visually in front of you (on the blackboard) and transfer it down onto paper. The coordination of the visual with the cognitive gets disrupted. You're constantly looking up, looking down, and you can't get it, as hard as you try.
GD: It wasn't a matter of simply just doing the task. Many of these suggestions imply, "Just do it!" This is the experience of many of these children. Their parents said, "If you just listened to me and just did this or that, things would be better."

Alexis: Since you're very very hyper, I wonder how you get your homework done.
Therapist: Alexis, how do you get yours done? You're an active girl.
Alexis: First, I have a lot of candy, then a lot of chocolate milk.

MN: I don't think that'll work! (Laughs) A sugar high!

Therapist: Wind yourself up even more! For real, what do you do when you're that active?
Alexis: I go outside and roller blade and go on my bike, and do sports, and go to my neighbors.

MN: She was also raising an interesting point. The roller-blading gave stimulation to the entire body and afterwards she had experienced that was able to calm down.
GD: That's a remedy for many hyperactive children. Alexis had received occupational therapy, so it was nice to hear her integrate those ideas into her daily life.

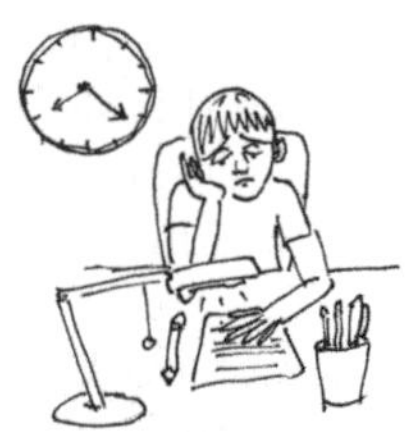

Boys' Group #3

Justin: All you need is some concentration and you'll be able to do it and be happy with your life. I have ADHD and I'm doing just fine. Concentration. Putting your mind to it is the trick.

MN: Was Justin medicated? He doesn't sound like he was.

GD: No. His mother sought more homeopathic remedies such as dietary changes and provided Justin with occupational therapy to help improve his attentional problems.

Therapist: Do you have any ideas on how to do that, Justin?

Justin: Hmmm. Tell yourself, loud, strong, and clear.

Leo: Two pieces of advice for you about your ADHD. Contain your after school energy by joining the track team or soccer team or whatever. And second, about the cleaning the room part. Get a maid!

Jamie: First of all, get to your house and try to see if you can play outside for about 1/2 an hour. Run around like a crazy squirrel if you need to get out all of your energy. Second of all—the bedroom cleaning thing. Just do it! I have the same problem with my bedroom. Believe me. I get to relax on weekends somehow. And if it's really getting on your nerves, lead your mom to court. End of story.

MN: This group was charming and very funny. It was very boy. There was a sequence here that is interesting. Leo is talking about "containing" energy, but actually what he was talking about was focusing your energy. Jamie was talking about aimless release which was much less functional. These comments were related to each other.

GD: Both of them were bringing in the mother—"get a maid" "lead your mom to court."

MN: The "lead your mom to court" would perhaps be for the crime of not understanding.

Therapist: Jamie, your idea of having 30 minutes to run around and get your energy out is really helpful.

Oliver: Well, I kind of know what it's like. My room is not really messy. I have to get up at 6:00 in the morning. Set your alarm for 5:30 or 6:00, clean your room and do all that stuff and you'll have enough energy to keep yourself awake in the day. Also, try to learn two things at the same time. In math class, I listen to the teacher and read my book at the same time. I'm doing that to be accepted at my school. It's hard, just keep at it, man.

MN: I don't understand that—doing two things at the same time. With ADHD, a person can barely do one thing, although sometimes background "noise" such as the radio or TV being on but not-really-listened-to can somehow help the youngster focus on the single task-at-hand. I've never understood why that is.

GD: I was also puzzled by his idea of doing two things at once, but I didn't want to distract the group by focusing on this sidebar issue. I think that what happened for Oliver was that he had little self-awareness and he did not claim his ADHD. I'm interested that he offered his comment right here, probably as a way of being accepted by his peers.

MN: There was a bit of a false-self at work here as well: trying to do two high-concentration things at the same time. This is not often possible for a youngster with ADHD unless it's to have the television in the background to do your homework. He was talking about reading a book and doing math at the same time and that's truly unrealistic. I agree with you; he was trying so hard to be accepted by the others in the group.

GD: It underscored his sense of being excluded by peers in general and his belief that there was something "wrong" with him.

MN: He did include a useful suggestion: setting your alarm clock early. The messy room issue reminds me of a youngster who had to clean his room once per week in order to collect his allowance. His mother told him, "And don't forget to clean the surfaces." He was nine years old and he asked, "What's a surface?" He couldn't find one. She said, "It's that flat thing that's beneath the underwear you left on your desk last week!"

GD: It's at times like this that it really helps us to realize that their world is such that they don't see clean surfaces. It's not something they even perceive.

MN: It's very similar to what their dressers look like. Everything in every drawer—just go and even try to find a pair of clean socks!

GD: No order at all.

Therapist: That's really good advice.

Jamie: A thing about the homework. Before you leave everyday, write yourself a note in a ton of different places on your desk. Ask the teacher what the assignments are or ask her to write it down for you. Make sure to bring your books home. If you're still remembering your assignments, hopefully you won't forget the books, too. If you can't do the homework, either destroy a few books or get yourself a stress ball. There! I destroyed a cup!

GD: He was! He was shredding a cup during this discussion. I wasn't sure if the destruction of the cup was his agitation about this letter, reflecting how hard this was for him or discharge of energy.

Therapist: You boys are really showing a lot of care for Adam.

MN: I think that was true. Once again, this group was demonstrating both their capacity for empathy and the openness to be touched by the letters. Here, I think Jamie's also saying that he was angry about his condition that he wished he didn't have it. "Damn it! And look, I even destroyed a cup right now."

GD: The cup was a plastic cup and it wasn't an easy thing to shred. He even used his teeth to make it happen. His anger about his condition was so clear!

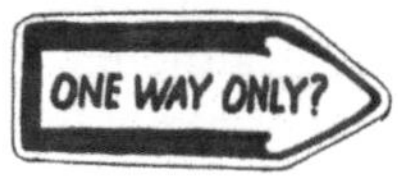

Boys' Group #1

Henry: I don't have ADHD and I can't relate so I can't help this time. Sorry.
Jacob: I have it. My mother says I don't have it, but I do. It's annoying to have it.
Therapist: How is it annoying for you, Jacob?
Jacob: I have to do extra stuff that occupies time.
Therapist: Are you saying that you're active? (Yes) How are you active? Everyone's different about being active.
Jacob: I always like to move.
Javier: I don't have ADHD. I have something—an extreme boredom disorder. I get bored incredibly easily. If I'm sitting doing nothing, nine times out of ten, I will get so bored, I don't even pay attention to something that might not be boring. I just get insanely bored.

MN: He was not talking about an attentional problem. He was talking about boredom. Sometimes boredom is defense against something else, such as anger, sadness, or frustration.

Therapist: So what do you do?
Javier: I don't do anything. I just wait until whatever it is will be over, like math.
Duncan: Well, Adam, you see. You forget a lot of stuff like writing down the homework. I say, actually my mom and my other relatives say, that I have a photographic memory. Which I do. I remember things about my life several years ago. The only thing that I do have a lot of trouble remembering is things about school. At school I have a lot of trouble remembering. I actually am pretty active when I'm at home.
Henry: There are some ADHD kids that I do know. Instead of them writing down their homework, we have planners at school. They write it down for them.
Therapist: That's a good suggestion, maybe he needs that.
Aaron: Does anybody have ADHD in here?

GD: As he was saying this, he was tipping his chair back.
MN: Tipping the chair back suggests to me that he was literally trying to get his bearing and, metaphorically, that he wanted to feel grounded emotionally by getting this information from the group. He then would know where he stood; he could then be on the ground level with the others.

Therapist: Is it important that we share that information?
Aaron: I have ADHD.

MN: He didn't want to be the only one with the condition.
GD: And several of the boys were saying that they didn't have it. He was feeling his differentness.

Therapist: What does that mean for you, Aaron?
Aaron: Actually I have more than that. But I'm not going to say it.

GD: He had bipolar disorder as well.

Therapist: You don't have to say it. Say only what you're comfortable saying.
Aaron: Actually, I like saying it because I like getting out of my body. I like getting everything bad.

GD: I wasn't sure what he was referring to. I was confused.

MN: I like this piece because it showed how the therapist could get confused and not be able to make sense of what was being said on the spot. With the safety of hindsight, I'd guess that he was trying to say that although he may have appeared really out of control, he did this on purpose. He might be claiming that he had more control than it may look to other people—when in fact he didn't. This was bravado to me.

Therapist: Are you active like he is?
Aaron: Yeah.
Therapist: How do you manage it? Adam (the letter-writer) would like advice on that.

GD: I took a re-focusing approach here.

Henry: I'm not very active. But even when I'm not paying attention, I still can listen and get information in.

GD: I think Henry was saying "that's not me, I'm not one of them!" He wanted to make that clear to the group. Henry might have felt, as so many people do, that even associating with peers with ADHD would cause him to develop ADHD. It is as if people feel that ADHD is contagious and that they could get it by maintaining close contact with someone who has it.
MN: These boys were really working with the identity issue. "Is ADHD part of <u>who</u> I am or a condition that I <u>have</u>, not really myself or part of my personality?" It's almost an existential question.
GD: I liked this process very much. I was hoping to elicit the meaning of what it was to have ADHD. And I was trying to do it as simply as possible.

Javier: Two things. One: sometimes, when I get really bored when I'm not doing anything, I have this tendency to not pay attention to anything. I'm bodily sitting there and my mind is not paying attention to anything in particular. My mind is in the void, the black hole. I'm looking for area of space where there is absolutely nothing. One piece of advice is that your school puts up a web site. My teachers put up their assignments there. Of course, they often forget or are late in doing it. It works when they do it.
Therapist: Some of you boys have learned something about each other today. I just wanted to share something with you about me. I don't have ADHD, but I definitely have an active body. More restless than a lot of people. I have to exercise everyday and if I don't, I fidget and I'm restless. Does anybody in here have that?

GD: I wanted to bring myself into the group process. I felt that I needed to after what Aaron had said. I think that self-disclosure is important at times.
MN: I agree completely, even though many people are trained never to self-disclose. Of course we have to be judicious about it, but often therapist disclosure can make a great deal of difference to our patients. They feel joined, rather than treated as "The Other."

Henry: I don't like moving at all. I just don't move any of my body.
Therapist: You're the opposite of me.
Javier: I can relate to that because I'm fidgety.

MN: Georgia, here's a great example of how your self-disclosures are facilitating the group process.

Javier: We go up to Canada every year. It usually takes two or three days just one way. I cannot stand holding still in a car for that long. (A boy yells out "Get a Game Boy!") I don't have a Game Boy.
Jacob: Get one of those cars with a DVD!
Javier: The problem is that we stay up there for a month.
Jacob: Get an R.V.—a house that moves around on wheels. It even has a basement.
Javier: We bring tapes, music, story tapes, all sorts of things.
Therapist: Why don't you stop every hour and get out and move around?

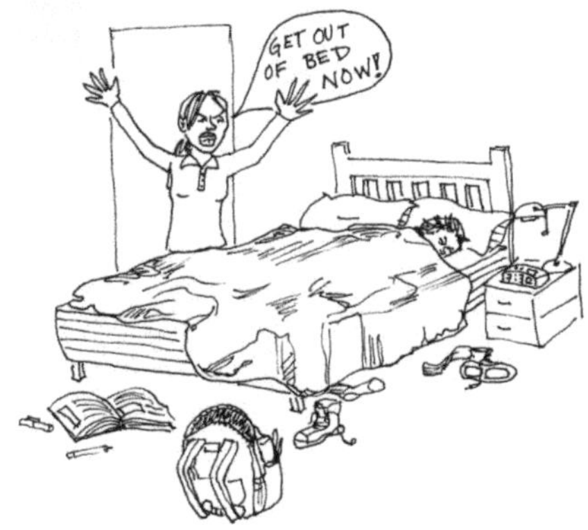

Suggested Activities

1. Design a perfect day's schedule. What would you do, when, where, and with whom?
2. True/false game: Tell something that happened to you in such a way that it is either a very fantastic tall tale or a bizarre story that really happened. Other kids guess whether the story is real or not real. Score a point for every child that was fooled. Children who guess correctly win a point.
3. Do a mindfulness activity. Use hand lotions with different scents to touch and smell; an interesting visual prop like a bubble column to look at; or a wind chime to listen to. Concentrate all your energy on this one thing. See if you can push all other thoughts out of your mind and focus only on the thing you are seeing, hearing, or touching right now. Do this for several minutes and see if you can calm your body and mind. If there are distractions, what are they? How does your body feel when you are doing only one thing at a time?

References

Brown, T. E. (2005). *Attention deficit disorder: The unfocused mind in children and adults.* San Antonio, TX: Harcourt.

Levine, M. A. (2003). *One mind at a time: America's top learning expert shows how every child can succeed.* New York: Touchstone Books.

Sommers-Flanagan, R., & Sommers-Flanagan, J. (2002). *Problem child or quirky kid?* Minneapolis: Free Spirit Publishing.

CHAPTER **8**

“What’s Wrong with Me?”

The letter in this chapter explores the theme of understanding how children make sense of their own special needs. It was written to evoke questions such as “What’s wrong with me?” but also to highlight the ways that many children may use their diagnosis to rationalize some of their behaviors.

A youngster might genuinely believe “my ADHD made me do it,” or she may consciously use her difficulty as a rationalization for some other problem or misbehavior. The letter was written to help evoke material from the children so that they might make the shift from reifying their diagnosis (“I *am* my problems”) to seeing their problems as only part of who they are as human beings (Bandura, 1997; Barkley, 1997).

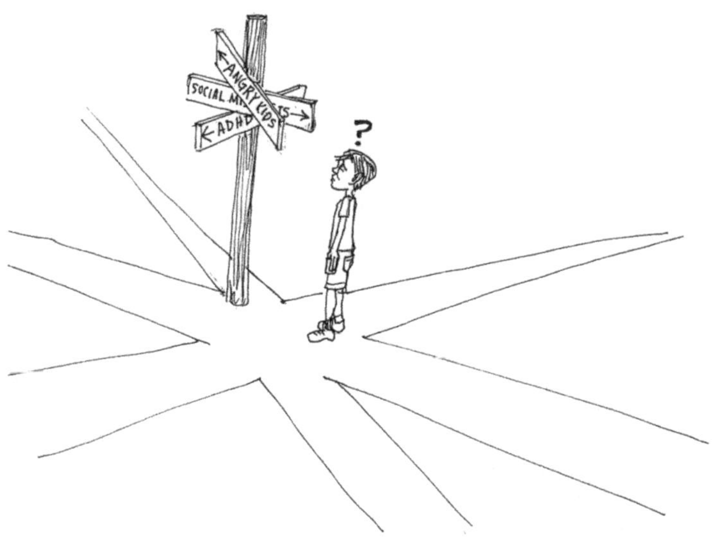

Dear Kids’ Club,

I think that there is something really wrong with me, but I don’t know what it is. It’s got to be pretty bad because I see a lot of different doctors, tutors, psychiatrists—you name it! As far as I can tell, I must be really stupid and completely checked out for me to need all these people. Nobody tells me what is wrong with me. I sometimes worry that it might be something like a brain tumor or that I'm really retarded and no one is brave enough to tell me. Whatever is wrong, I can't tell that anything is getting any better when I go to see these people. Besides that, it's a lot of appointments and that takes away almost all my free time.

All I can figure out is that I hate school and that it is really hard. I read things and they fly right in and out of my head. So when the teacher asks questions like, "What was the main message of the story?" I completely glaze over, duck my head, and hope that she doesn't call on me. My teachers don't seem to like me, and so far this year I have absolutely no friends. The only kid who plays with me is that little kid who is 3 years younger than me who lives down the street. I don't really understand all this and wish that I could move away or even run away and start new someplace else. Maybe that would solve it. Then I would have a fresh start and "the problem" I have will disappear. What a relief that would be.

Do you have any ideas what could be wrong? How can I find out?

Signed,
Pete, the Puzzled One
(Penny in girls' version)

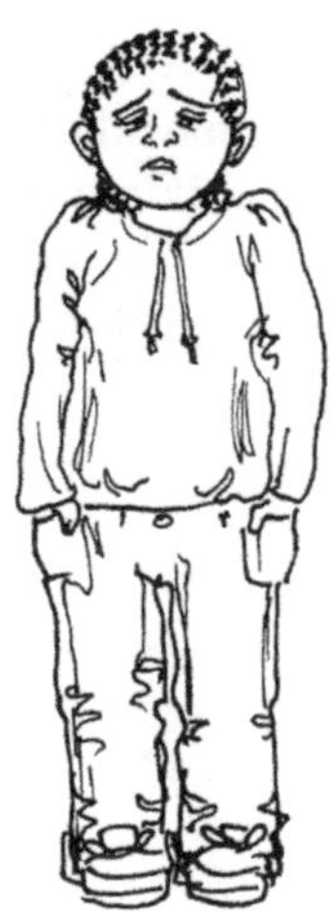

Boys' Group #3

Oliver: It still won't solve your problem. You can't run away from your problems. Also if you're afraid that you might be retarded, well, my teacher last year—she had a best friend who was mentally retarded and he apparently is a millionaire. So even if you have a problem, just get through it. When I was born, I also had a problem. It's not the same as yours, but I could have died from it. That's why I'm able to blow my nose a lot. Last year with that same teacher, I got into problems a lot at school. This year I'm like the best kid in the class. So starting over is the right thing, but don't run away. Get a clean slate. Pretend you're in a new place. That's what I did. Try to make a good impression. You'll probably come out the same way. Keep that, man!

GD: He was referring to reconstructive esophageal surgery that he had when he was born. Oliver changed schools last year which helped him get a fresh start and a chance to be in an environment where he wasn't pegged as the geek or outcast like he was in his last school.

MN: Wouldn't it be lovely if Oliver could have appreciated some of his special qualities: his thoughtfulness, capacity for empathy, and healthy sensitivity. It might have helped mitigate his self-loathing and fantasies of self-harm? This made him an especially good candidate for group therapy because feedback from a group represents the power of peers. The clinical dilemma was for the therapist to truly "know" the group and therefore know whether to say something to Oliver or not. Would the group have been able to sustain Oliver or not? Here was an example of when it was important that the therapist say something, as an inoculation for Oliver, just in case . . . .

Therapist: That's so empathic and excellent advice, Oliver.

Leo: Just because you don't have a lot of tutors doesn't mean that anything is wrong with you. I have a physical therapist and I used to have a private tutor. Everything you said is something I can relate to except for the fact that you have no friends. I have one friend, a friend. Even this thing, this group, is a physical therapist. All this stuff that my mom gets are books about the coordinated child. It's not done squat for me. Actually looking at all of us in boys' club, saying that isn't much of a consolation.

GD: Leo started out saying something quite empathic and helpful, then ruined it at the end. This was what he did all the time in the course of any interaction. He was a very likeable boy, and then he would do something outrageous. I was worried that his insult about how the group looked would have had a negative impact on the group process. Jamie acknowledged the comment with an "OK," but dismissed it and moved on.

Jamie: OK.

MN: Jamie managed this group-moment very well. He handled Leo and got the group back on a more productive track.

Jamie: My best advice for you to do is for your learning problem. Read a lot of books which will help you. Also, if you need a friend, the best thing to do is help somebody and they will look at you as a friend. Or get a dog if no one is nice to you.

MN: The dog comment was both sad and sweet at the same time.

Justin: If you see a real lot of doctors and tutors, demand to know why you're getting so much help. Demand, demand, demand!

GD: Justin was struggling to understand himself and was hungry for information from adults to help him. He was very brave and intelligent, and had an excellent capacity to integrate information about himself without feeling demoralized or overwhelmed. For example, he always wore ear plugs in group when the noise volume got too loud for him. He simply accepted this as a quirk about himself. He would say things like, "I have sensitivity with my hearing and this is what I need to do about it."

MN: He was a good example for the other boys in the group. Those group members who used group by learning vicariously would have particularly benefited from

Justin's attitude about his problem. A quiet group member can still be an active group member by the quality of his attention. Some children use this way-of-being in the group very productively, learning vicariously from the discussion. It's interesting how, in most groups, such a member is accepted as truly a part of the group.

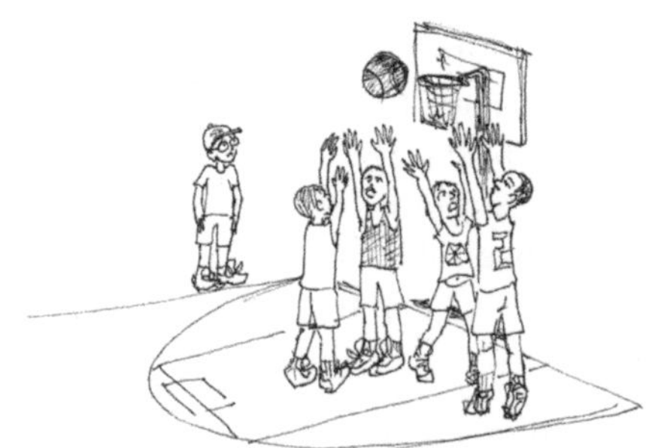

Boys' Group #1

Henry: Welcome to my world. I know exactly how you're feeling. I went to a doctor once who said that I was retarded, autistic, and had ADHD. He said all those things about me from just meeting me a few times. I remember going home the night that I learned I was retarded and I cried into my pillow all night. I thought my life was over. My parents fired the psychiatrist who said this about me because none of it was true. I discovered that my learning style is different than other kids. I happen to be a person who needs time to come up with my ideas so I look slow to other people, but I really have a lot of intelligence. It was very difficult when I was going through all this. The thing that has helped me has been having things like this club and some tutors who helped me learn that I really didn't have retardation or autism. I do have some ADD problems but I am learning to manage this.

GD: What a heart-felt response to this letter! I was so struck by the internal pain that Henry struggled with over the years in learning that something was wrong with him.

MN: I'm struck by how much he trusted the group.

GD: Henry was the boy who was told that he was participating in an experiment by coming to our group, so I wondered how the group became safe for him and when he began to become more honest and forthcoming. He was also speaking about how he appeared to others. Even though he was very intelligent, he was aware of how "slow" he looked to others. His slowness was a function of his low muscle tone and passive motor style. He was quite content to sit and often looked flat or expressionless. After Henry's admission, the group became chaotic and disorganized. They could not handle his emotional pain and engaged in various antics like tipping over chairs, poking at one another, and generally falling apart.

MN: Sometimes this sort of thing happens in groups when one child discloses too much, too fast, and the other children relate too much to the material, then have to back away because it is too close to home for them.

GD: Henry was very vulnerable on that particular day. I remember we ended up doing a group construction project gluing wood pieces and corks and molding shapes with clay and Model Magic™. Henry seemed very anxious until he settled upon making a structure that looked like a large phallic looking rocket ship coming out of a launch pad. He kept saying, "I have no idea what this is." I inquired calmly, "Well, take a guess. What could it be?" He continually said, "I have no idea," so I replied, "Whatever it is, it looks very powerful to me." This is a good example of how useful it is to follow the letters with activities that provide the group members an opportunity to explore their feelings through projective activities. It can be very organizing for the children on both a verbal and non-verbal level.

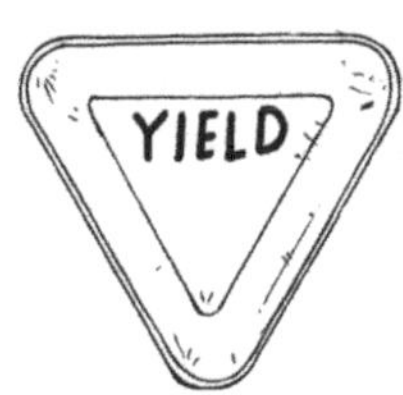

Boys' Group #2

Ian: Pete. I feel the same way. I don't even know why I'm here, but what I'm saying is, try to be friendly to other people. Study a lot. You could even make some new friends if you tell them the truth. And about the psychiatrists and people, ask them why they're there. Or ask your parents. That's my advice to you.

Kevin: How long has this been going on? He might try asking his parents to let them know that he really cares about this and is interested. Ask them and don't accept any excuses. He's probably not suffering from any disease. I call this reverse psychology. You think you're suffering from something, and you don't know what's going on. It also depends on how many times he is he going to the doctors and psychiatrists because if he's going twice a week, once a week . . . .

MN: Something about his comment was bothering Kevin. His last comment was incomplete and it's meaning could only be hypothesized. His language became defensively obfuscating and therefore communicatively incomplete. I would guess that the discussion about "being different" had become too much by this time.

Ian: At school there are all these adults being a little too nice to me. It's a type of nice where I get treated better than the other students.

Aidan: That's called accommodations.

Therapist: Are they doing extra things to help you out?

Ian: Yeah. Accommodations.

Therapist: That's not a bad thing, Ian, to have accommodations to help you out with your learning.

Kevin: So when he's in school and one thing goes in his mind and out of it, it matters. If he's losing his attention and letting it wander. I had that problem a bit and my mind wandered. Now I concentrate more and listen to the teachers more carefully.

Aidan: If you're feeling this stressed and have this kind of problem, tell your parents, "I have the right to know what's going on with me so I can solve my problems easier. If you're keeping them from me, that'll be more difficult for me. They're my problems. You're going to let me know what they are so that I can solve them myself. Not just you solving my problems."

GD: He owned his problem and had come to grips with what it meant to have ADHD.

MN: I like what you did here. It's something that, as therapists, we don't do very often. You offered a value judgment when you said, "That's not a bad thing." You were letting him know your personal opinion: that it wasn't a terrible thing. This interaction speaks to the therapist needing to be aware of when to share a value judgment. There are other times we may not do so because it could stop the group the process. In this instance, the group needed your opinion, because it was validating of their group interaction.

GD: I knew that Ian was not seeing a therapist for individual work, so I wanted to find a way to put validation into my response.

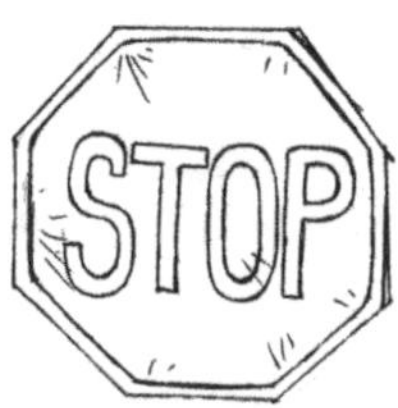

Girls' Group #5

GD: Brittany submitted her own letter to the girls' group. At that point over the course of the groups, the youngsters wanted to write letters, often anonymously, to the group for feedback. Occasionally they wanted the letters to be read in other groups to protect their anonymity even more. Here is an example of one letter written by a girl in the Girls' Group#5. One of our ongoing group therapeutic goals was for children to open up to others about their concerns and about their lives.

MN: Yes, and from a therapeutic point of view, this desire to write their own letters was a demonstration of how what we do in group continues in the patient's mind between sessions. The therapeutic "action" does not just occur during the group sessions themselves.

GD: And so Brittany carried us in her mind.

Dear Girls' Club,

I try to tell my friends and family that I don't like myself but nobody understands. I thought maybe you girls would get it and give me some help. Everyone who knows me just says that it's silly to dislike myself because I'm so nice. They also say I should think about all the stuff I do well and how many friends I have. They don't realize all that doesn't change my mind.

When I do something well or get a compliment, I only think it won't happen again or that someone is just trying to cheer me up. When I like someone at school, I try and try to get her to like me even when I can tell she doesn't want to be best friends. Then I feel so mad and hurt that nothing works. I even forget about my old friends sometimes because I'm always trying to get a popular girl to be a new friend.

I don't understand why I can't like myself and just think of what's wrong with me. Sometimes, I think I will do something even I don't expect that makes me unlikeable and everyone will hate me. I'm beginning to not want to go to birthday parties because I'll find out the girls like each other but not me. Help me please. I don't want to stay this way.

Signed,
Diane, feeling Desperate

GD: I saw Brittany in individual therapy and helped her to write this letter because of her problems generating a coherent written piece.

MN: Did the group know she wrote this?

GD: No. She wanted to protect her identity, so she gave the author of the letter the name, Diane, feeling Desperate. The girls didn't know it was Brittany.

Brooke: Why do you think you hate yourself? I know you might think you hate yourself but think about all the things you love to do and how good you are at them. Just try your best and figure out why you hate yourself and make a chart. Show your mom.

GD: She concretized this, and made it too simple.

MN: And in some ways she recapitulated the letter-writer's experience, which she had already said was unhelpful.

GD: She also tried to distance from the feelings of self-loathing that the letter-writer felt by saying, "Make a chart."

Brooke: Tell your mom that you need help in liking yourself. Ask her "What's good about me? What's to like about me?"

MN: This was a little better. Brooke was getting closer to a combination of problem-solving and self-examination.

GD: Yet she recommended asking others to reflect on what could be good about her. It was possible that she couldn't bear to think about her own self or if she did look within, what she saw was not a good reflecting image.

Brooke: What I have to say is that you shouldn't hate yourself from what you look like or what you are. You should hate yourself from how you act. You should like yourself for who you really are. Maybe your outside can be really ugly, but the inside is not. Most of the time they're both really nice, so good luck.

Brittany: I feel like that some days. I sort of get over it at the end of the day because I talk to my parents about it. But sometimes it may not work when you talk to your parents about it. Talk to one of your closest friends. Tell them about your day and ask them about how they feel about their day. You'll probably feel much happier.

Therapist: You know what I was thinking, Brittany, nobody likes everything 100% about themselves. Most of us like a big part of ourselves but there are some things that we don't like so much. You might like—(I elicited from the girls in the group) your art, your heart (generosity), your creativity, your soccer playing, being a sweet and generous person, your sense of humor.

Brittany: My mom actually makes me happy because she tells me really funny jokes when she e-mails me. I could tell one. My mom e-mailed me this one joke—What happened to the 2 peanuts walking thru the bad neighborhood? The answer is "One got assaulted." So it makes me laugh sometimes. Also this e-mail that a relative sent. At the end the dog was laughing so hard because the cat was wet. First step was- put the cat in the toilet, second step- flush the toilet. The cat lives. At the end it says, your toilet will be nice and clean and so was the cat.

MN: I'm not sure what provoked such a peculiar comment, and it was coming from the person who wrote the letter. It seemed so disorganized.

GD: All I could think was that she was regressing before my eyes, and feeling terrible.

Therapist: What you're bringing up is that we can distract ourselves from bad thoughts or bad feelings by laughing. That is one way. But we still have to take care of the fact that we worry about not feeling good about ourselves and how we can feel better. We need to keep talking about that in here.

GD: I wanted them to know that we were going to keep working on this issue.

MN: These concrete ideas, which were not really bad ideas, didn't really go to the heart of understanding why someone hates herself. I would want to keep this issue alive, especially as they got older and continued this self-loathing. I would not want them to do that and would worry about the eventual development of self-harmful behavior such as cutting.

GD: It was not surprising that in the groups we've discussed in this chapter that this issue of "What's wrong with me?" touches a raw nerve with many of the children. We saw several groups where the children fell apart or regressed in some form. Again, it points to the importance of when one opens up emotionally charged material, how the therapist needs to "put the group back together" again through validation and activities that restore the children's emotional equilibrium.

Suggested Activities

1. Draw a mandala on a circular piece of cardboard (cake pan size). A mandala can be any design that the child constructs from their own imagination—abstract designs, a picture of hands overlapping one another, or any design of their own making. An alternative activity might be to present the child with a piece of paper with an empty vase outline and see what the child draws inside.
2. Group appreciation: Each week the group leader can choose another group member for the children to say what they appreciate or like about that child. Write it down for them to take home.

References

Bandura, A. (1997). *Self-efficacy. The exercise of control.* New York: W.H. Freeman.

Barkley, R. A. (1997). *ADHD and the nature of self-control.* New York: Guilford Press.

CHAPTER 9
"Jumping Out of My Skin"

Many children with learning disabilities, attention-deficit hyperactivity disorder, Asperger's syndrome, and mood-regulation problems experience sensory hypersensitivities. Children with *full-spectrum Asperger's syndrome* typically exhibit a combination of learning disabilities, serious social mis-attunement, attention-deficit hyperactivity disorder, sensory hypersensitivity, and difficulties with affective dysregulation (Klin, Volkmar, & Sparrow, 2000). Parents and professionals often misunderstand these difficulties, especially regarding how the sensory problems impact relational dynamics (DeGangi, 2000; Miller & Fuller, 2006). There are some children, for example, who have *motor planning* problems coupled with difficulties in *executive functioning*. Such a symptom constellation makes it difficult for that child to understand how to be with peers or how to generate and persevere in group games or activities. Children with *auditory hypersensitivities*, on the other hand, often cannot tolerate the level of noise that is typically generated by groups of children having fun, for example, in noisy environments like the playground or lunchroom. If the child has *tactile defensiveness*, he is apt to be overly reactive to being bumped or touched by other children. The tactually defensive child often misinterprets friendly touch as aggressive. In contrast, some children may seek out heavy touch contact with peers because of a *under-reactive tactile system* and be viewed by others as aggressive when in fact they are craving physical contact. Children with *sensory integration* problems are often treated by an occupational therapist to address how sensory underpinnings relate to self-calming, better attention, organization skills, motor planning, and functional learning and motor abilities. Unless the youngster works with a mental health professional who understands sensory integration processing disorder, the child may not understand the connection between sensory problems and his experience of emotional distress or social difficulties. This week's letter relates some of the typical experiences of a child with problems within this realm of development.

Dear Kids' Club,

I am a really sensitive kind of kid. When I say sensitive, boy, do I mean sensitive! I hate being touched by anybody. If my mom or dad tries to give me a hug, it makes me feel like jumping out of my skin. If a kid bumps into me at school, it feels like a cinder block knocked into me. I think that kids know I have this touch sensitive problem because I don't wear any socks no matter what time of year it is, I roll my shirt sleeves up all the time, and I can only stand really loose clothes so I don't exactly look like everyone else in the clothes department. There are days that I swear kids purposely bump into me because they know it gets me so upset. One day last week I pulled out my sharpened pencil and held it out at arm's length prepared for the next time anyone tried the *bumparama* on me. It got me into big trouble because I poked the point right into some girl's back. She started the whole thing, knocking that backpack of hers into me about 40 times in a row.

The other thing about my sensitive nature is that I can't stand too much noise. The lunchroom and gym drive me nuts, all that echoing of kids yelling and shouting. I have to press my fingers tight into my ears sometimes, or I just bolt out of the room to get away from it. Sometimes I just yell out "QUIET!" but then before I know it, everyone is yelling at each other to "SHUT UP!" The teacher grabbed my arm the other day when I did that and said that I was "out of line." Of course, her grabbing my arm set me off, and the next thing I did was punch her in the arm. That was the day I got sent home from school.

Does anyone else in your group have this kind of sensitive situation in their body? I think the best solution is for me to become like that Bubble Boy who isolated himself in a special air tent in his house. That would work wonders for me. What do you think I should do?

Signed,
Bill, Bubble Boy's Twin Brother
(Betsy in girl's version)

Girls' Group #4

Caitlin: If somebody touches you, turn around and say, "Could you please stop touching me because I don't really feel comfortable." Also say, "Please be quiet because I'm trying to do something."

Therapist: That's nice how you use your words instead of popping pencils into kids or yelling. Does anybody in here have a touch problem?

Caitlin: Sometimes I touch my friend, Julia, and she doesn't like to be touched.

Therapist: So you know somebody who doesn't like to be touched.

Caitlin: She says to me, "I don't really feel comfortable about that."

Therapist: Anybody sensitive to noises in here, like the gym or cafeteria noise?

Caitlin: Well, the fire alarm bothers me because it's so loud, like a loud Tweety Bird whistle.

Therapist: And that bothers you, Caitlin?

Caitlin: Yeah, because I have to cover my ears like this. (Demonstrated.)

MN: Caitlin was describing herself. She was responding to, but not yet verbalizing, an empathic connection to the isolation described in the letter. She was in problem-solving rather than feeling mode. However, her contribution was better related to the real topic and better organized than sometimes her responses tend to be. She said, "Can you please stop touching me because I don't really feel comfortable." It had a soothing quality to it. "Please be quiet because I'm trying to do something." She does understand the problem, and if I'm hearing the tone right, it was quieter and softer than is typical for Caitlin.

GD: This was probably the most related Caitlin had been to a letter. It was a specific symptom that she was talking about, and she was able to relate to it. It was very body-oriented and that's why she sounded better.

Hannah: I don't really like noise. It just gets too noisy for me in the cafeteria and I can hardly hear the kid next to me when we're talking. It's really noisy. It takes a while for the teachers to get the kids to quiet down. It's really annoying.

Therapist: So do you like it when it's nice and calm and quiet? Anybody have advice for Betsy.

MN: The safer aspect of the non-sexual body-oriented problems is keeping the group process going. Caitlin can be more related within the group, and Hannah can pick up the group issue and continue the work. I do wonder what Hannah meant by "annoying." Some children become infuriated with other children because of the imposition of noise. Others blame themselves for being so different that they can't handle what other kids manage very well.

GD: Sometimes, a youngster with Asperger's or other types of learning disabilities may take her reaction so far as to misperceive other children as purposely trying to annoy her by being noisy, and perhaps even making fun of her by doing so.

MN: It's a persecutory interpretation of the situation and a good example of how youngsters with Asperger's have a mis-attuned "theory of mind." They cannot correctly understand the intentionality, interpersonal behavior, and thinking of others. The letter-writer was using aggression as a way of controlling what's going on.

GD: So many children with tactile problems use aggression as their way of coping. Adults sometimes misinterpret this, in an unintentionally but nevertheless unempathic way. That's why I wrote this letter. Children like this are misunderstood and very isolated.

MN: You're really talking about the regulatory attempts children make as well as the response of the environment to them. The letter-writer was tactually defensive and what could he do about it? It was not going to go away and he knew it; instead, he tried to regulate his environment. However, his attempts to deal with this problem were not helpful. There was more that these girls could have responded to in the letter. For example, how did they know that something was wrong with the way they experience touch or sound? They were aware that they were quite different than the other kids around them. There is then a risk, especially for children with Asperger's, for social avoidance to increase and become crystallized as a social maladaptation.

GD: Many of these children have such distorted sensory perception that it alters both the ways in which they think about their own emotions as well as their ability to filter affective responses.

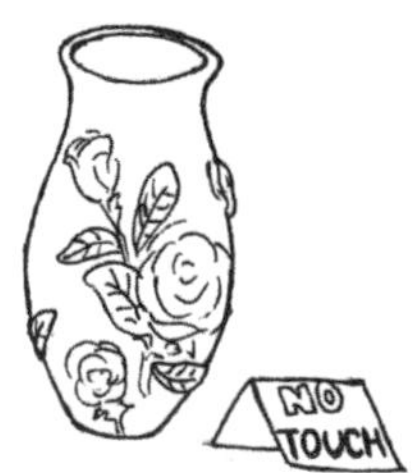

Boys' Group #3

Therapist: Bill, here is the Tuesday boys group. When I read the letter to the group, there were several boys here who were spontaneously raising their hands and saying, "That's me!" So here's Justin.

Justin: I was one of those kids who was sensitive but at least to sound. Boy, do I notice things! I wear ear plugs. Sometimes I run out of the room. I was in a class that was GTLD (Gifted and Talented/Learning Disabled), which was supposed to be tailored to my needs. Sound often gets me. Maybe you should get your mom a psychologist for this, for the sensitive part.

Leo: Psychiatrist! (Whispers to Justin)

Justin: Psychologist!

Leo: Psychiatrist!

Justin: Psychologist! (Even louder) All right, let's just hand this off to Oliver.

MN: That was a nice way of having the last word and getting the rest of the group involved at the same time. It was almost elegant.

GD: And what I liked was that they identified that a professional such as a psychologist was needed to help them understand what it means to have this problem and how it impacts their social relationships.

Oliver: I don't really have this problem but I could say something. I don't have any experience with this so I don't really know.

MN: Is that true?

GD: Yes. He was the only boy in the group who did not have sensory integration problems coupled with social and emotional problems. His problems included a good does of anxiety with depression.

MN: Oliver's failure, then, to "say something," even when he says he could, is interesting within the context of process. Justin had handed the ball to Oliver. Oliver then withheld that "something," as if he were annoyed with having been put in the "speaking position" involuntarily. As a therapist, you had a choice to make: pursue the letter-writer's issue because it was so close to the group members' experiences, or to work with Oliver's feelings in the moment. You made the decision to help Oliver speak to the letter-writer's experience.

Therapist: If you were a friend of his, what would you say to him?

Oliver: I'm being serious about his touch thing. Try to ask your family to help you. Have them keep on poking you until you get used to it. Then try adding different kinds of touch. If you have a brother or sister, try to have them actually hit you. That's what siblings often do. When you get used to it, the touch thing will be resolved. And for the sound thing, try fighting fire with fire. Buy CDs and crank them at loud volume. Try and try to withstand it, just like with the touch issue. Eventually your problem should be solved. It may take a while but face it!

MN: He didn't understand because it wasn't his experience. Nevertheless, he was making an attempt at being helpful by recommending desensitization, even if his ideas were in some ways unrealistic. He was also trying to address the letter-writer's sense of helplessness by making a suggestion that has a large degree of self-instrumentality.

GD: He assumed that this problem could have been corrected by just facing it. In a way, though, his idea about how to approach the problem was courageous.

Therapist: You know what you're saying is something called desensitization. It's something that therapists teach kids to do. Bingo! You could have my job!

Leo: Bill, if that is your real name. Ba-ba-boom! I have a case like you, but not so extreme. I was never sensitive to sound, but I couldn't stand tags or wearing a sweater with nothing under it. I still can't do this—wearing a shirt with buttons on the inside.

Therapist: I know a lot of kids like that. They have to wear button-free clothes.

Leo: Buttons on the inside are a no-no. Every Monday I went to an occupational therapist and she did gymnastics and stuff. On the bar there was a scooter board where I would lie on my stomach and smash into bean bags. Somehow that actually solved my problem. I think you should try to get an occupational therapist. The answer is exercise with bean bags!

GD: After the group, Leo came up to me and gave me a big hug and seemed very relieved. He used to smash into other kids, poked pencils into other children, and did similar annoying behaviors. I think he felt good talking about this in the group and being acknowledged or validated that this was a legitimate problem. The boys did understand what the letter-writer felt. This sequence in the group showed that there could be almost a confessional kind of relief just in talking about something.

MN: The letter itself may have given Leo the sense that, indeed, he was not alone. There was someone else out there who was like him. There were even kids out there he didn't know who have this problem.

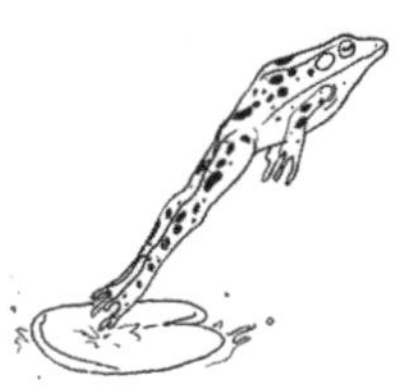

Boys' Group #1

Jacob: I only have the hearing problem that you have. I can hear loud noises and really can't stand echoes in cafeterias.

Therapist: What's your advice?

Jacob: I leave as soon as possible.

Therapist: Suppose you are in a situation where you can't leave. How do you handle it then?

Jacob: Sneak out.

Therapist: So you take a break like go to the bathroom or something?

Jacob: (no response).

Henry: I saw this kind of thing in a book and I heard about it in the news. It's a weird condition and this girl had to wear gloves and stuff when she ate dinner. Her parents had to watch her because if she touched something with her hands, she would freak out and have like a seizure. I don't know how to fix it or the sound problem. If you were in my school in our cafeteria, you would go nuts. It's really loud. The teacher has to wait 5 minutes after she says "Be quiet" and it's still loud. Some people have this reaction and act really strange after it.

MN: Jacob and Henry both perceived the environment as failing to be helpful, but not purposely so. The environment can't realistically provide the support that children need, in a timely fashion. This letter evoked the interaction of the supportiveness of the environment to the child's own experience and that the environment could have done some fixing of it, like getting it quiet. These youngsters weren't quite ready, but in a few years, hopefully, they would be able to understand that developing coping skills for their difficulties was going to be necessary because there weren't going to be other people who could or would intervene so readily. A time will come when they will have to use what they've learned when they were younger in order to know how to manage on their own as young adults. This is another reason why early treatment is important, and that these boys were essentially receiving a gift. They also were fortunate to have been specifically in group psychotherapy so that they could learn strategies from the other group members, understand that they're not alone, and hopefully have memories when they are older of what they learned from the other group members.

GD: But the fact of the matter is that the children in metropolitan areas such as New York, Los Angeles, or Washington, DC may experience greater distress from their problems of sensory integration than children growing up in the hills of Wisconsin or Vermont. The combination of the city environment, its pace and noise, as well as the sheer population size, would make that true.

Therapist: Anybody have this problem with the touch or sound and have advice for Bill?
Javier: Sounds like you have a big case of claustrophobia.
Therapist: I never thought of it that way.
Javier: Claustrophobia. It has to do with closeness of a sheer area.

MN: I think he was saying that his auditory sensitivity caused him to experience ordinary sounds as amplified noise.
GD: As if he were in an echo chamber.

Therapist: Have you ever had that yourself?
Javier: Not often and it only happens if I'm in a really crowded area.
Aaron: I'm claustrophobic in here.

MN: It's interesting that Aaron inserted this comment here, within a small group. I think he was ready to express his discomfort with the content and that the group was still able to stay on-topic. He was attempting a (failed) defensive maneuver to shift the topic. "Claustrophobic" in this context was a metaphor for "this is getting too close for comfort." Again the therapist was confronted with the need to be able to identify metaphorical communication when it is occurring and then decide how to use it. In this instance, you retained faith in the group process to override the potential defensive shift that Aaron attempted. The group rose to the occasion and kept going.

GD: Something was bothering Javier too. It was noticeable in the quality of his next comment.

Javier: When kids bump into you, the best way to prevent is not to react. You do something to them and it gets you in trouble. No teacher is going to buy that, "They bumped into me on purpose." If they do, they have to be able to prove it and of course, they can't. Don't do anything because it only gets you in trouble and it doesn't stop the other kid from doing their thing. I used to have OCD—obsessive compulsive disorder. If I touched something accidentally with one hand, I had to touch something with my other hand in the same spot because it didn't feel right. It doesn't make any sense at all, but that's how it worked.

MN: That was an idiosyncratic response and I find myself working hard to try to understand it. In the moment, during the session, this comment would have given me pause. Javier was being very practical but his response was off-kilter, almost tangential. In the room, I would start to wonder, "what's bothering him right now that his thinking has shifted so markedly?" He's stopped really keying into what the youngster in the letter is describing.

GD: He was concentrating on not getting in trouble. He was concentrating on the behaviorally oriented and moving away from the internal experience of what it felt like to have these problems.

MN: So, in a way, and hearing this in retrospect, Aaron's comment really was an expression of the group zeitgeist and not a purely individual attempt at defending only himself from uncomfortable content. This is a good example of how fluid the therapist needs to be in understanding the ever-changing content, level of communication, defenses, and whether those defenses are in the service of the ego (serving a stabilizing function in this case) or in need of interpretation as maladaptive. Hard work!

GD: It's interesting that he merged obsessive-compulsive disorder (OCD) with this letter—like a compulsion to touch versus a sensitivity to touch. The interaction of the group dynamics seemed clearly related to the constitutional difficulties these boys had. They were emotionally sensitive at that moment, vulnerable, and it was showing in the group process. It became clear when their feelings about their physical vulnerabilities were playing out in the group.

Therapist: That's helpful that you're sharing that, Javier.

Javier: It was a fairly mild case, but was a problem.

MN: Nice recovery.

Tyrone: I don't have much of claustrophobia and I get that way in an elevator when it's really tight. Sometimes I think that I won't be able to get out in time.

GD: I didn't know he had claustrophobia in small spaces. But I did think that Tyrone was picking up on the group's anxiety or group claustrophobia at facing these body-related problems in themselves.

MN: It's possible that he was getting anxious and feeling that the emotional group tone was "closing in" on him. He wouldn't be alone: Aaron and Javier both expressed their discomfort although each in his own style. He said he didn't have that problem and then he proceeded to describe that exact problem. His anxiety might have altered what he was going to say in the first place. It's an example of anxiety disrupting language.

Henry: The thing I'm saying about kids bumping into you at school is done a lot to make kids feel really bad. Like they bump into you to make you drop all your books and then everyone can laugh at you. It's called trucking, whacking into someone at really high speed.

Therapist: They do that a lot at your school?

Henry: Yeah, it happens every few seconds. It's a normal way that people walk in the hall because it's so crowded.

GD: Henry had a problem with being whacked or "trucked" into at school. He was often picked on in this way.

MN: He was also not responding to the problem in the letter but to his own experiences. What it felt like to be picked on is not really in the letter. Nevertheless, Henry was talking about his sense of victimization. That was the connection to the letter: implicit feeling rather than manifest verbal content.

GD: I often think about when there is a true language problem that is causing a secondary anxiety and when there is primary anxiety that is causing a secondary expressive language disruption.

Aaron: First of all, when you said you hit your teacher that was probably your biggest mistake. If you hit your teacher, you're in big trouble. I know that because in third grade, I hit my teacher a lot and ended up in the principal's office every day. There's got to be a consequence from someone of higher authority than you.

MN: He was pulling the group back on course. He had recovered from his earlier discomfort.

GD: And even though his comment did not relate directly to Henry's comment, both boys are disclosing times in their lives when they were either the aggressor or the target of aggression.

Henry: If your mom and dad know about this, they should be telling the school about it. The school nurse should know it by now. It's not easily solved.

MN: Again the group expressed the need for useful environmental support. This may also have been a description and recognition that the group was working very hard.

Therapist: You're bringing up a good point, Henry. Bill may have to live with this for a long time, perhaps his whole life and he'll have to figure out how to manage it.

GD: This is the reality of many children with sensory integration disorder. They are not always going to have the opportunity to rely on environmental support. They need to become more instrumental in handling their problems so that they can manage better as adults.

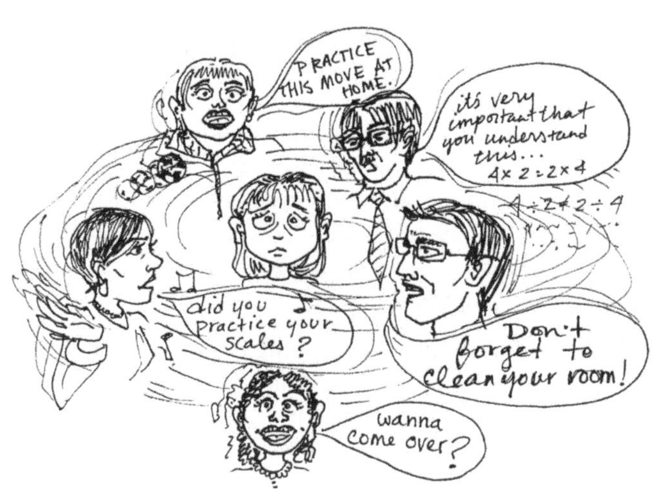
PRACTICE THIS MOVE AT HOME.
its very important that you understand this...
4× 2 = 2× 4
4 ÷ 2 ≠ 2 ÷ 4
did you practice your scales?
Don't forget to clean your room!
wanna come over?

Suggested Activities

1. Using the sensory profile, interview the children as a group to discuss what calms them down, revs them up, and sensory activities that they seek or avoid.
2. Using pieces of colored tissue paper, rip or cut them into random shapes and place them in a aluminum cake tin. Add water to the tissue paper to create a tie-dye effect. When the project dries, children can make the tissue paper design into a picture to frame. As children engage in this project, the therapist can comment on how the child does the project. For example, do they use a lot of water to blend colors or do they cut precise shapes versus more random ones? The project can offer a window into the process of how the child organizes an open-ended project of this sort.

References

DeGangi, G. (2000). *Pediatric disorders of regulation in affect and behavior: A therapist's guide to assessment and treatment.* New York: Academic Press.

Klin, A., Volkmar, F. R., & Sparrow, S. S. (Eds.) (2000). *Asperger syndrome.* New York: Guilford Press.

Miller, L. J., & Fuller, D. A. (2006). *Sensational kids: Hope and help for children with sensory processing disorder.* New York: Putnam.

Your Sensory Profile

	Like It	Avoid It	Find It Calming
Auditory:			
1. Loud music	____	____	____
2. Soft relaxing music	____	____	____
3. Playing a musical instrument	____	____	____
4. Humming and singing to self or others	____	____	____
Visual:			
1. Dark places	____	____	____
2. Bright lights	____	____	____
3. Lots of colorful things around you	____	____	____
4. Wearing colorful clothes	____	____	____
5. No clutter in sight	____	____	____
6. Things organized in their places	____	____	____
Movement:			
1. Rocking in a chair	____	____	____
2. Swinging	____	____	____
3. Jumping on a trampoline	____	____	____
4. Roller coasters	____	____	____
5. Being high off the ground	____	____	____
6. All kinds of movement rides	____	____	____
7. Sports, dancing, or exercise	____	____	____
8. Falling	____	____	____
Touch:			
1. Messy art projects	____	____	____
2. Getting a hair cut or washing hair	____	____	____
3. Wearing fuzzy clothing	____	____	____
4. Being barefoot	____	____	____
5. Being in water, taking showers or baths	____	____	____
6. Getting touched by other people	____	____	____
7. Touching or hugging people	____	____	____
8. Doing projects like knitting, clay	____	____	____
9. Wearing tight clothing	____	____	____
10. Wearing loose clothing	____	____	____

	Like It	Avoid It	Find It Calming
Mouth:			
1. Crunchy foods like pretzels	____	____	____
2. Eating spicy foods	____	____	____
3. Putting things in your mouth to chew on like gum	____	____	____
4. Smelling certain scents (cinnamon, lavender)	____	____	____
Joints and Heavy Work:			
1. Exercising	____	____	____
2. Lifting heavy objects or doing weights	____	____	____
Activity Level:			
1. Quiet, sedentary play like watching TV, reading, and computers	____	____	____
2. Active, on the go activities like hiking, bike-riding, and sports	____	____	____
3. Having a busy schedule	____	____	____
4. Prefer a lazy day with not much to do	____	____	____
Social:			
1. Looking people in the eye when talking	____	____	____
2. Being around lots of people in a crowd or a party	____	____	____
3. Being in quiet places with only one or two other people	____	____	____
4. Laughing and joking	____	____	____
5. Having serious conversations	____	____	____
6. Working on projects as a team	____	____	____
7. Having alone time	____	____	____
8. Changing routines or having new things to do	____	____	____

What Things Do You Need To Do for Yourself to Feel Calm and Organized?

1. Sound stimulation____
2. Visual stimulation____
3. Movement____
4. Touch____
5. Joints or heavy work____
6. Mouth stimulation____
7. Active things____
8. Social stimulation____

PART II
Interpersonal Effectiveness

Interpersonal effectiveness is the focus of Part II. These letters section address problems related to social problem-solving, working with others collaboratively, decision-making, developing leadership skills, and being able to participate in conversational discourse in social groups. The "Dear Kids' Club" letters in Part II aim to facilitate the fostering of children to become able to understand problems of impulse control, sharing control with others, and developing flexibility in social interactions. The letters also address such common problems as being excluded, rejected, or teased.

By the time the topic of interpersonal effectiveness is brought up in the course of the group's life, the group should have become cohesive and able to work productively, using its process. At this stage in the life of the group, the children should have developed more self-awareness of the problems in their lives and of what obstacles they have in developing friendships. Often children who participate in groups such as these struggle with reading social cues, have limited insight into the nature of their problems, and difficulty understanding the perspective of others. These children are apt to jump to conclusions or see problems in concrete terms, overlooking the nuances of social situations. In addition, they are likely to experience developmental challenges such as poor executive functioning, difficulties with pragmatic language, and social misperceptions that make conversations and interactions disjointed. Their attempts at conversation are often hard for others to follow. They may also have developed a variety of defense mechanisms to help them at least try to minimize their distress and to rationalize their behavior (Klin, Volkmar, & Sparrow, 2000; Hall, 2001; Siegel, 1999). Part II of the book explores all of these issues as they manifest in a group therapy setting.

CHAPTER 10
Living with a Short Fuse

The first letter in this chapter is in the voice of a child who is himself the bully, rather than the bullied. He faults others for his own shortcomings and has an all-too-easily–activated temper. The letter-writer expresses a common lack of insight into his own behavior and is unaware of how his actions have an impact on other people, including peers.

> *Dear Kids' Club,*
>
> I didn't really want to write this letter, but Georgia made me do it. So, I'm pleasing her. Here's the deal. I get in fights all the time at school. Last year, I was suspended twice for calling kids really bad names and cursing (in boys' version: for giving someone a knuckle sandwich). The kid totally deserved it. She/he was making wisecracks about my jacket, and if she/he weren't so stupid all the time, I wouldn't have to keep telling her/him what to do. I have to say, "Get your butt over here and stop yakking." The kid irritates the heck out of me and on the school bus, I feel like knocking her/his lights out. It's the way she/he looks, her/his goofy laugh, and her/his constant talking. If she/he would get a life, I wouldn't have to keep her/him in line. Someone has got to do it, so I guess it's my job. Georgia thinks that I have a temper problem. Maybe I do, maybe I don't. I also get mad at my stupid little brother who's always in my room taking my stuff. He deserves what he gets. And I have to admit, I call my mom some serious names ("you stupid bitch") when she orders me around. So I did what Georgia told me to do and here's the letter. If you want to say something in my defense, that would help.
>
> **Signed,**
Adam, Really an OK guy
(Alicia in girls' version)

GD: I wanted to incorporate the issue of resistance into this letter. This child has no clue that he is a big part of the problem or that he resists accepting responsibility for any part of his problem with anger management. I wanted to create the tone of a bully who blames others for his own misdeeds. It is easy to picture this child's meanness to others.

MN: Yes, this is a kind of child that all of us has known. As with many bullies, there is an utter failure of empathy. He doesn't understand the extent to which he can be creating his own problems, or at least exacerbating them. He also hasn't any idea of his effect on others, the hurt he renders.

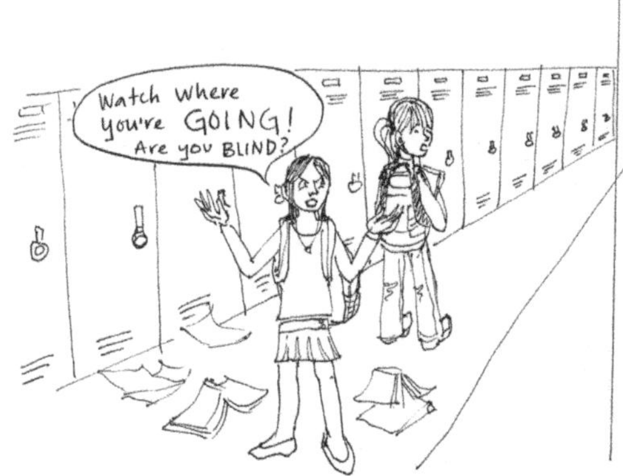

Girls' Group #3

Alexis: She's stupid.

MN: Therapeutically, this comment called for the therapist to pre-empt a group descent into name-calling and to bring it back to the relevant issues in the letter.

Therapist: You know, she's going to hear this.
Alexis: OK, I take that back.
Gillian: Alicia, I know how you feel, because I get into really big fights. I learned this from my dad. You could use this. Hug, hug, then you talk about what's going on. Then you could just say, "No more brothers bothering me." Is there something that I could do? Well, Georgia's the one to talk to. Sometimes I get into big fights with my brother and when I come see Georgia, I talk to her about it and she makes it all better. Now I know what to do when I get in fights. Either tell my mom or dad or whoever takes care of me.

GD: She passed the buck to someone else by not owning the problem.
MN: To me, this had to do with not looking for help. The content of Gillian's comment had to do with making the problem someone else's responsibility.
GD: And not owning the anger that's within. That's the toxic nature of anger. It makes them want to get rid of it.
MN: I worked with an adult in group therapy for several years. He was a very angry person and ashamed of it. During one group session, I sat on the table in the middle of the room and asked him to shake my hand. He did, but then he tried to pull his hand away. I kept holding on tight. He started to look angry at first, and then really scared. I said, "I will let go. Tell me what you feel." He said, "I'm scared." I said, "What are you scared of?" He started to cry and said, "I will infect you." I knew that in some ways I was breaking the rules about touch, but I had been working too hard to find a way to help him reach this material. I also had

confidence in the strength of the therapeutic alliance or else I would never have attempted such prolonged touch.

GD: How interesting that he thought he would pass his anger into your body and infect you with it.

MN: He might have felt, "I am so angry and so filled with this poison, that I will kill you just by having contact." I mean that phrase as a metaphor for the level of his pathology in interpersonal relatedness.

GD: I hear that a lot from the adults with whom I work, who say that their anger is poisonous, toxic, and it's pulsing in their veins. They want to get rid of it. They worry that it will destroy the people around them.

MN: Some of this dynamic was occurring within this girls' group.

GD: Many of these children were so angry that they needed a therapist to tolerate the distress of anger experienced by the child and sit with the emotional tone, to bear it with them. It's what Winnicott called "containment" (Winnicott, 1965).

MN: This includes tolerating your own counter-transference response to someone who is provocative. You do feel angry back, but it is not toxic to you, as opposed to the fear and toxicity that your patient may feel. It is not toxic to you because you have accepted that experiencing aggression is simply part of feeling human. It's a very powerful concept to help the group start to understand. And it certainly is one very difficult task!

GD: They were clearly avoiding talking about it here. Nevertheless, I tried to nudge it along in what I said next.

Therapist: Does anybody else get angry sometimes and do things that they regret later?

Kendra: When I was six, I got really angry and kicked my wall and my foot got stuck in the wall.

Therapist: You broke a hole in the wall?

Kendra: Then a year later we got a paint job and fixed it.

Therapist: Since then you haven't kicked walls?

Kendra: No, I haven't.

Therapist: I was just wondering. Have you all figured out that everyone gets mad? It would help Alicia to hear about you girls, what happens to you when you are angry.

Alexis: I get mad at my horse sometimes. Sometimes he's in a really bad mood and won't eat. I get mad at him and he ends up eating the grass.

Therapist: What do you look like when you get mad?

Alexis: I don't know.

MN: She concentrated on the stimulus—not on herself. She wasn't responding to what you asked, "What do you look like when you get angry?" and ended up with the horse eating grass. It's an escape mechanism at work: flight/fight. This defense also commonly operates on a group level.

Deborah: If you get mad at somebody, don't do anything to them. Imagine that you're tearing them into tiny little pieces and throwing them against a wall and dropping them off buildings and stuff. Just *imagine* that you're doing that to them. That makes you feel like you really did it.

Therapist: Deborah, you frequently think of things to use in your imagination.

GD: I liked Deborah's response very much. It showed some thoughtfulness and her intensity told me that she really felt what she was saying.

MN: Yes. I'm interested in how the rest of the group responded to that comment. There was no pretending here, no smoothing it over.

GD: She was the only one in the group so far who was willing to face the anger.

Ashley: There's this girl who really annoys me and when she does something and the teacher hears it, I think "This is really nice." She gets in trouble all the time.

MN: She's giving you a bit of sarcasm. I think this was a defensive maneuver because the material troubled her.

Elizabeth: This is like Deborah's idea. What you could do is copy pictures that are faces and when you get mad, then tear their face up. Like you're tearing their life apart.

GD: I was surprised that Elizabeth came up with a strategy to direct her own anger. Her typical response in group was not to respond or to reply: "I don't know." She was quite avoidant of her feelings.

MN: She picked up on the intensity. Should I assume that she could live with this idea?

GD: Actually, this wasn't really in keeping with how she usually responded.

Therapist: That reminds me of voodoo. What would it look like if we were sitting in your bedroom and watching you have a tantrum?

Ashley: I don't know what it would look like. I never do that unless it's with my sister.

Gillian: I look so angry (big sneer on face). I yell and Georgia can actually know all this because I see her alone sometimes and I tell her all about my anger.

GD: She needed to pull me in. Gillian often lorded it over the other children that she got individual time with me that the others didn't. It was aggressive toward the other girls and she meant to create envy. It was hurtful.

Therapist: I just want to say one thing about anger myself. Sometimes when I'm mad I want to yell or kick things or hit things because I'm so bursting. Then there are other times that I'm so angry and furious, I have the opposite response and just want to cry. It depends on what is making me angry.

Alexis: When I get angry, I go downstairs and I tackle my dog. He doesn't care. I hope I don't kill him one day.

MN: She was obviously worried about her aggression getting out of control. Her experiencing aggression as toxic was palpable.

Therapist: He doesn't mind when you jump on him like that? Girls, I know that Alicia didn't want to write that letter. Alicia, I hope these comments help you out.

MN: There was a sequence to this particular group session that is very interesting. Many, even most, group sessions have an arc. Something is defended against within the group, but then the group gets down to what really matters and they talk about it with real feeling and intensity. Then the group process, often toward the end of the session, will bring the emotional level right back down to the defensive part where it began. I think that's a good way to end the group and return everyone to emotional safety. We can see this particular dynamic in this session really nicely.

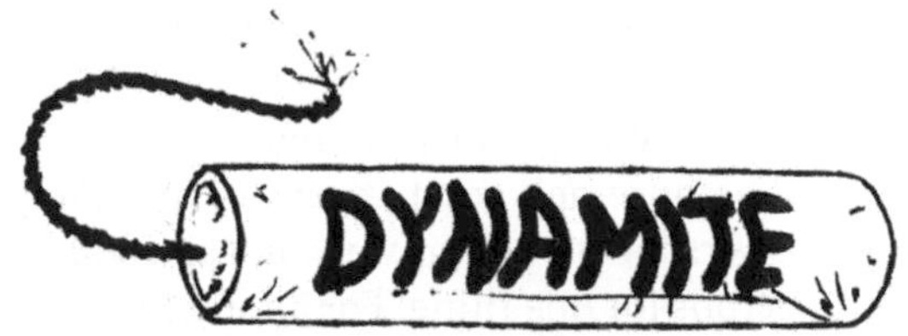

Boys' Group #3

Justin: You're probably a pretty normal guy. Sometimes use words instead of names or questions, so tell your mom. You have to do what she does. You can't survive a long time in your life without your mom. One more thing—debug. Ignore them, talk to an adult, walk away if he keeps yakking. If an adult doesn't listen, you've got a big problem.

MN: I am so confused by what he was saying. Are we still talking about the letter about the bully? The use of computer language—"debug"—is appealing, though.

GD: Yes! This didn't follow at all. I think he might have been trying to offer the "debug" rules that schools teach to protect against bullies. I was quiet because I wanted to see if the group could keep the focus by itself. Leo did bring the focus back.

Leo: I'm sorry about this, Adam, but I think it sounds like you're really a bully. Just give the poor kid a chance. Boys club, I'm speaking to you. He probably won't believe me, because I'm the kid who gets bullied around a lot. It would really help me if you backed me up. Adam, you shouldn't order him around all together. When he annoys you, just get away. Do something else on the bus, like read a book or listen to your Walkman™.

GD: I was so proud of Leo for speaking up. This was one of the few times he spoke of his own vulnerabilities at being the bully's victim. He also addressed the letter-writer directly by making a plea to think about what he was doing. Leo knew first hand how painful it was to be the target.

MN: He made it clear to the group what they were really talking about. I had lost track myself after what Justin said.

Jamie: Some advice for your little brother. Get a lock to your room. And also, have a few spare keys in case you ever lose your lock. And also, for that annoying kid at school, when he annoys you on the bus, get a Game Boy, play it. Or just doodle on the bus. And also, I have a question for Leo. Leo, how can you get bullied around? You're kind of big to be bullied around. Use your weight advantage.

GD: Jamie was offering ideas as if the boy in the letter could understand them. I like that he turned to Leo and showed his surprise that Leo didn't look like a bully. That was validating to Leo that he didn't have a bulls-eye branded on his forehead ready for the bully's target practice.

Leo: I'm like an average kid. Most kids are at least as tall as me. Some bullies are just a few inches shorter than me. And they're much stronger than me.

Therapist: Is that part of the problem—they muscle you around?

Leo: No, they just whack at me when I'm not suspecting. I made friends with one of them, Tommy.
Therapist: That's good to know. That might help Adam.
Leo: It actually started because he's good at science and I'm good at math. We give each other the answers for the things we're not so good in.
Nate: Keep away from gerbils for one thing. For another thing....

GD: Nate was very upset by this discussion.

Therapist: Seriously. What would you suggest that would be helpful?
Nate: For one thing don't use that language, or else. And....

MN: It's to Nate's credit that he allowed you to try to bring him back.
GD: Nate would be extremely bothered by a child bad-mouthing his mother. He was very attached to her and used her to keep himself soothed and organized. She was a very caring, nurturing mother who managed to remain calm in moments when Nate fell apart. I could see that he was struggling with what to say.

Therapist: Take your time.
Nate: Don't take it out on him; take it out on the patrols.

MN: He came up with an unhelpful response, using a displacement defense. The boys were struggling with the issues presented in the letter and we can see that in the unevenness of the group dynamic. It oscillated between being on-topic, then off-topic, then back to on-topic. This dynamic was, in essence, both portraying and "betraying" the boys' discomfort.

Oliver: First of all with your little brother getting into your mom, you should save up for a special lock. It's like a spy lock. That annoying kid. I kind of know what it's like to be that kid, except my case is more extreme. There's this one kid who is the target for one thing. I'm just saying this to you from that kid's point of view. Mine is more extreme. At lunch if anyone sits next to me, they're considered infected.
Therapist: That's horrible.

GD: Oliver was not the bully. He was the recipient of merciless teasing. He would hold his emotions inside and somehow think that what's inside spills to others who merely sit next to him at the lunch table.
MN: We're seeing, in this group too, the belief that anger is poisonous and can "infect" others.

Oliver: I'm telling you this from that kid's point of view. Try to see it from how he sees it and what it would be like.
Nate: Keep away from bee-bee guns.
Oliver: Nate, that's not helpful.

MN: Good for Oliver, a good example of functional group process: self-correction.

Therapist: Look at Oliver. How do you think he's feeling right now?
Nate: Well, it's true that he should.
Therapist: Oliver is telling us something that is really upsetting to him.
Oliver: As for your telling all that bad stuff to your mom, try and make some kind of a swear jar. When you swear, you put change in there.

Therapist: And if those kids at school who were doing that thing to you, if they did that, perhaps that might make a difference.
Oliver: I don't think so. When I was in soccer and I was trying to get a soccer ball, they said, "Get out of them before Oliver gets them." I really don't like it.
Justin: Introduce them to me and I will take care of them.
Oliver: They're just going to think you're mean and take it out on you.
Therapist: Oliver, I think Justin is really trying to be on your side.

MN: Justin was really trying to help. Oliver, however, was looking for strategies to handle these problem situations himself. They are recurrent and someone coming to his rescue isn't a long-term solution. Nevertheless, it's so touching that Justin wanted to help him.

Oliver: What I'm telling him is . . . (sigh).

MN: As so often, Oliver was a real heart-tugger.

Therapist: Justin, are you saying that you really want to help Oliver, and if you could go to his school you would be by his side? That's very supportive. Leo, earlier, you were saying that you were the one who gets bullied. This is a similar kind of thing but with a different twist on it.

GD: I tried to pull the group process together by summarizing the key points of their discussion to keep the focus.

Oliver: Yeah, I never can bring in sugary snacks. I just bring in FruitLovers™. They say that I'm some kind of freak.
Therapist: Justin is very upset that he's hearing this happens to you.
Justin: Can you explain exactly, clearer to me, Oliver?

GD: Justin was continuing to react with such empathy and warmth toward Oliver. He was able to sustain it. In my comments, I was also trying to help the children to read one another's cues.
MN: And he was addressing Oliver directly. Instead of the group relying on the therapist to be the "hub" of the group wheel, the "spokes" (the youngsters) were addressing each other. This is a powerful group process, but very hard to sustain. Often the therapist has to become the hub again.

Therapist: Do you want to say anything more about this, Oliver, because Justin is very agitated that this happens to you?

GD: I continued to reorient the group to Justin's obvious agitation. I didn't want to let this go—both to help Justin in feeling better understood and to help the group members to refine their signal reading and to respond empathically in a helpful way.

Oliver: After school if I want to play a game with them, they say that the only way I can is if I do a lot of stuff for them, like find five pine cones in less than ten minutes.
Therapist: Like being a slave for them.
Oliver: Even if I do that, they say, "go do this, go do this" and finally I do a lot of stuff, then I say, "I don't want to do this anymore."
Justin: Maybe try to find a day when there is somebody in your group who actually wants to play with you. Or you could subject them to what you've been through, and do it even more harshly

MN: Sweet revenge.

Therapist: That's the instinct. When somebody is really horrible to you, you want to get them back. An eye for an eye.
Justin: I mean I want them to know how it feels to have this done.
Therapist: What do you think, guys, if Oliver says he's going on strike and won't do these things anymore?
Oliver: It won't solve anything. It would just continue.

MN: His helplessness was palpable.

Therapist: I think in this group we can take Oliver's problem and role-play it and come up with ways to handle it. Would that help you out?
Oliver: I think it would help, but the really interesting thing and seeing the Misfits play at our school a few years ago, some kids were seriously taunted a lot. The only way they could get out of it was to go to school with guns and shoot the kids. Or people commit suicide.

MN: This comment is very concerning. It had the potential to disrupt the group because of how extreme it is.

Oliver: There's a kid at school that said that there was a person at his dad's school who was taunted so much, that one time he went home and committed suicide.

GD: Interestingly, Oliver did not express these dark thoughts with his individual therapist. The opportunity to express himself in a group setting, and in particular with these letters, provided him with the displacement that he needed to verbalize what he was feeling inside.
MN: He wanted the pain to stop, and so he identified with people who had truly physically hurt themselves.

Therapist: Have you ever had that thought yourself?
Oliver: No, but I have done some serious thinking about trying to go to a new school.
Therapist: That might be a good solution to the problem. It's not something that you have to just sit with. You can also try to do what Justin said, to try to find some people who actually want to be with you.
Oliver: I doubt that anyone wants to be with me.
Therapist: Look in this group here, Oliver. You have a lot of support in this group.
Leo: I'm with you.

GD: During all this, Jamie was drawing a picture of action figures shooting at one another and then showed it to Oliver. He was very frightened by this discussion.
MN: I think Jamie had actually been empathizing, but not in a healthy way. He seems to have identified with Oliver's pain, but dealt with his experience by getting involved in aggressive, perhaps vengeful, fantasy.
GD: I worked hard to use the group process to help Oliver become able to take in the gestures of support that had been offered to him. He was a very intellectual child and preferred to interact on a verbal level. Even when he was being showered with positive gestures of support, he didn't seem to take it in unless I helped him to notice it. At the end of the session, Leo handed me a letter he had written on the sly during the session, about his being bullied at school. He whispered to me, "Can we make this be our letter next week?"

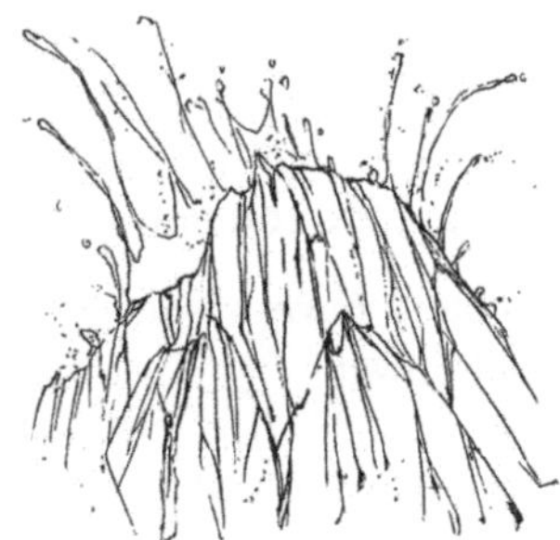

Boys' Group #1

Javier: The most scary thing is that you think that this is normal.

Jacob: Usually some kids can be very annoying like that, just ignore them. Most people say that, but it never works. Another thing, do something like that when no teachers are looking, and that's hard to do.

MN: Devious, actually, but it certainly wouldn't solve the problem. He was avoiding the feelings in the letter and not articulating his own.

GD: Jacob would try to sneak in impulsive behaviors when nobody was looking and then acted innocent when kids spoke out to the teacher about him. He constantly struggled with impulse control.

MN: Are we seeing the interaction of a constitutional factor (impulsivity) with an intrapsychic one (quick-trigger use of avoidance)?

GD: I think so. The coupling of the two yielded a child who lived alone with his feelings. It can develop into a pattern whereby the child lacks self-insight, ends up blaming others and the environment for his feelings and misdeeds, and a lack of mindfulness of others or the ability to take perspective.

Javier: My brother irritates me all the time.

Henry: I have this kid with ADHD in my class. I think he has something worse than that because he's annoying and runs around and shouts. Everyone deep down inside wants to whack him. Nobody does it because we don't want to get in trouble with the teacher. Try to refrain from whacking everyone.

GD: Henry was bringing up a reason for why the child might act this way. "Perhaps he has ADHD and can't control his behavior." But he nicely brought in the response of others to annoying behaviors.

Javier: My brother drives me crazy in the most extreme way. He drives me crazy about everything. Literally. I can hardly stand to be around him, even in the few times when he's all right. There is something that is bound to go wrong and we end up in a royal yelling match or argument. I never, ever play any kind of competitive game with him, especially Monopoly or a board game. I start winning, he immediately yells, "You cheated. I quit!" The whole 9 yards and it's all garbage.

Henry: I think it's natural for a little sister or brother to be annoying. My sister, if she sees that she's losing, she starts to act sleepier and lays down in front of the TV and throws pieces at me. Usually brothers and sisters are annoying and there's nothing you can do about it because they're younger than you and still developing. Your mom is still going to encourage them to be developing and in this case, annoying you.

MN: This was rather cute. The "experts" were expostulating. I think they were trying to express their sense of mastery.

GD: And what they've done is conveniently depart from the letter's theme, to being annoyed by younger siblings. The content of this letter was overwhelming them.

Jacob: Younger brothers and sisters have a special power called "mom power" and there's no way to beat that power.

Duncan: Or until your parents die.

Javier: Hopefully by then you will have moved away or your younger brother and sister will have matured.

GD: The group dynamic is really great here. The boys brought themselves into it and related their conflicts with their siblings in particular. And then they also described how they would get pulled into the battles. However, they tended to put the blame on their siblings, for the most part and not acknowledge their own contribution to the problem.

MN: This is a common position for boys this age to take. Seeing one's own part in problem situations involves losing face.

Jacob: For what you said about that person that always annoys you ....

GD: He trailed off and stopped talking. As I mentioned earlier, Jacob was the child who was most annoying to the others. There had been times in the group when I had to take him outside the group room because his behavior had gotten so out-of-hand and uncontrollable that he couldn't be managed in the room.

MN: Jacob's underlying mechanism might have been: "If other kids are going to reject me, then I will take control of the situation so I'll know when they'll reject me. I will become the Rejection Master." He seemed not to see his own behavioral contribution to his rejection by others.

Therapist: One of the things about Adam is that he flips his lid. How many of you have a temper problem? Three hands up, the hands are coming up. Those of you who have a temper problem, maybe you could share with Adam what you get upset about and how you handle it.

Tyrone: Sometimes I get angry when my friends don't agree on what I want to do. I always want it my way.

Javier: My way or the highway! You must rise above it!

Tyrone: I hate it whenever my brother doesn't agree with what I want to do, like watch the same TV show.

GD: The group discussion shifted nicely to the boys talking about their own need to have things their way and how their own inflexibility would get them into trouble with peers or siblings.

Therapist: What if Adam was here right now and asked, "What do you do when you try to do something smart and it doesn't work?"

Tyrone: I usually go crazy and sometimes I go along with what they want.

Therapist: One last question—are any of you the kid who gets picked on at school? If Adam hears the opposite side of the coin, what it's like for the kid who is picked on, that might help him.

Javier: How do you know that everybody else doesn't like this kid?

Therapist: He thinks that. He talks about this kid like, this kid stinks!

Javier: He can't read minds.

Aaron: Well, I'm somebody whose feelings get hurt easily so when somebody says something to me or didn't mean to hurt my feelings and they do. Like when we're playing football outside, I usually get picked last. Sometimes I can't catch the ball but that's not entirely true because people don't throw it to me and give me a chance. I used to be picked on more than that.

MN: This was not only insightful; it was from-the-heart.

GD: Aaron spoke so meaningfully about what it felt like to be on the receiving end. I was very impressed that Aaron brought this up. He opened up the group so that others felt able to speak about being picked on. His comments were poignant to me, too.

Henry: I used to be picked on constantly by one kid. I told the teacher and this kid got suspended. Now he doesn't want to go anywhere near me.

Tyrone: The person you're picking on may not want to tell the teacher or tell somebody and just because he hasn't told anyone, doesn't mean that you should still be picking on him. He could just be too scared to speak up. He might not know what other people might say if he tells on you and he doesn't know if you might come up and attack him.

GD: This was exactly how Tyrone would typically respond. I'm glad that he raised how defenseless and frightened the bullied child might feel. This group demonstrated a lovely sequence from the child who unknowingly sets others off with his impulsive actions to bringing in a topic that they could tolerate—annoying behaviors in others.

MN: They were then able to talk about how their own behavioral inflexibility could impact others while at the same time bring up how devastating it feels to be picked on. The group showed a level of sophistication in thinking by addressing the problem from these different points of view.

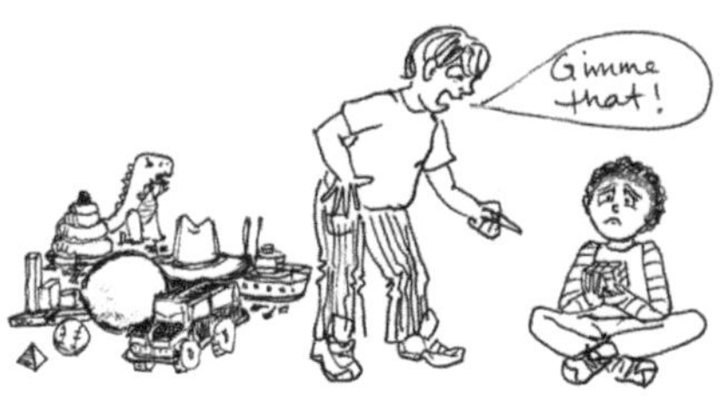

Girls' Group #5

Brittany: I have a relation to that. A girl in my class, Jessica, she tells some kids to shut up and she's like the boss of them, but she really isn't. She thinks she's in control of them, like she controls the world.

Brooke: I don't think you should call your mom that word because your mom is trying to help you grow up. Maybe if you just listen to her, she'll calm you down. Give her a chance. Your mom is not there to be yelled at.

MN: She was starting to be a bit pedantic, but that was just the beginning of her comment.

Brooke: She really doesn't like it.

MN: She then showed empathy with the parent.

Brooke: She probably feels like punching you right now when you say that to her.

MN: A bit of hyperbole but still on target, empathizing with mother's dislike of being treated with disrespectful disdain.

Brooke: I know my mom would feel like that if I said that to her. She'd put me in time-out. Never, ever, say that word!

GD: I was pleased that she was able to bring up the dynamic of the letter-writer and her mother because it fit Brooke exactly. She used to be very disrespectful to her mother and order her around constantly. This was a big problem that we had to work on. Her mother was able to remain calm and patient throughout the process of learning how to respond to Brooke. By this time in her treatment, Brooke was better able to keep her temper in check and talked through what frustrated her with her mom in a more reasonable way.

Nadia: Once me and my friend were fighting and I just told her to shut up because she kept getting in my face. She wouldn't listen so I just told on her. She said, "No I didn't." Then she tried to get me in trouble. Then when I went home, I had too much homework and I got really mad at my mom. Then I cursed at her. She got really mad at me. Then I knew that it was bad, but I did it.

Therapist: It's hard to talk about this stuff.

GD: Nadia articulated so nicely how the problem can start with someone else, like, in this instance, a friend at school who is fighting with her. She seemed to understand that she displaced her anger at the friend onto her mother.

MN: Actually, it was a double displacement: she displaced blame from her friend onto her homework (which probably shortened her fuse a bit), and from there onto her mother. Her awareness and articulation of the process of displacement served the group members by helping them, eventually, to see how they might also, at times, have relied on displacement.

Brittany: Violence is not the answer to solving problems. My parents taught me that. Also you could say bad words in your head and it may help, much more better. My mom gave me a punching bag and that works. It takes out all your stress and your anger.

Nadia: I break a pencil or punch a pillow.

MN: These comments followed nicely. They, too (the punching bag, pencil, and pillow) would serve as more adaptive displacement objects than another person. The girls stayed on-task; a nice process.

Melissa: About you're being really mean to your mom. I think that you should get some really good quality time with your mom. I do that with my mom whether it's taking a walk, folding laundry, or even stacking Oreos™ on the kitchen table. We like having time together after we've been really mean to each other. We try to make it even better. Sometimes even go out for ice cream.

Therapist: That's good. You're fixing the anger so that you don't end on a bad note.

MN: I liked the description of a reparation process between Melissa and her mother.

GD: When Melissa entered the group, she was having some horrible fights with her mother that centered on not getting her own way. Over the course of the fall, her parents worked diligently, spending "special time" with her, and providing her with focused, non-judgmental attention. Then when Melissa became agitated, they encouraged her to release her anger in productive ways and talk it out with them. She responded very well to these interventions.

MN: Yes, she was clearly showing how much she had learned. I'm glad you just described what the home situation was like; because we can see better just how well this youngster used her therapy.

Melissa: I think that at least if you curse, you should say, "I'm sorry, I didn't mean it." And talk to your mom about what's happening at school so then you won't have that much anger. Sometimes when I'm angry, I bang on my pillow.

GD: Melissa impressed others as someone who was completely incapable of expressing anger, so it was wonderful that she owned her anger and described how she expressed it.

Brooke: I think that your mom will make you feel like she doesn't want to be your mom anymore. (Note: Brooke was adopted.)

MN: This is sad; it's the bedrock fear of the adopted child. But at least she was expressing it.

Brooke: It will just make her cry. She cries in her head.

MN: I think she was talking about herself, her internal state when she would upset her mother, and perhaps her internal state in a less situation-specific way.

Brooke: If you do that again, you'll get in huge trouble. I don't think you want to go into that. Just stop doing it. Break a pencil or slam your head into the wall. Put glue in your hands. Pinch yourself when you do something bad. I used to do that. I would hit myself and pinch myself. Don't get in the habit of that though. I stopped. Try to think of something besides saying bad words to your mother. Your mom just tries to help you.

GD: Here is the self-loathing that occurs, especially in girls, when they experience anger. They don't always feel that it is socially acceptable to express anger and so they turn it inward to self-harm, like cutting themselves.

MN: I was thinking of Brooke as a potential cutter, too.

Nadia: Once when we came home from church and my brother kept being mean to me and cursing at me, I just kept saying, "Be quiet, shut up" and he said, "Make me." My dad got really mad at him because he was really tired of it. I didn't know what all this yelling was about. My dad was yelling at Sam so loud and pounding him on the floor. And I was, "Dad, can you stop it?" Then he stopped and Sam was being a baby.

GD: She's speaking about how difficult it is for her to tolerate anger from family members. Her last statement—that Sam was "being a baby"—makes me think that he started crying inconsolably after the fight and wouldn't listen to his parent's point of view.

MN: "Pounding him on the floor" suggests a lack of control on the part of the father. I don't know whether Nadia was referring to actual physical abuse or not, but this degree of anger, at least as she perceived it, would make it clear why tolerating family anger was difficult. On the other hand, if this was a misrepresentation of the facts, then we're seeing how Nadia's fear of anger distorted her view of the world. It would be an example of projection. This is an example of the therapist simply needing to wait and see.

Brittany: Once when I was really mad at my mom we both came in the house and we didn't say hi to my dad. My mom went into the opposite room and I went into my room and we both slammed the door at the same time. I felt like crying but I held it back. What I did was really wrong. My mom wanted to listen to the radio. Can you keep this a secret? My mom was embarrassing me. I said to my mom, "Can you please stop?" And she said, "So I'm not allowed to have any fun?" My dad yelled at her because she lost the pot lid. I turned off the radio, she turned it back on, and I turned it back off. Then she turned it back on and turned it down. After that we barely talked to each other. We did talk in the end. So spend some quality time with your mom or with anybody that you can. You're only a child a little while.

MN: This is very troubling. It sounds like this child's mother would start acting like a young child and join Brittany in a fight as if she were her sibling.

GD: Brittany often brought up similar conflicts with her mother and in each case, she worried about losing her. Her adaptation was to become parental toward her mother, trying to find ways to repair the damage. It's a very overwhelming task, especially for an adopted child.

Therapist: I want to ask the group something. Now, Alicia, I know that I said to you that you have a temper problem. Just so you know that other people have it, let's see a show of hands of how many girls in here flip their lids sometimes. Everybody has her hand up. Does that make you feel any better? I just wanted to say that there are different ways of flipping lids. Like slamming doors, punching pillows, breaking pencils. Sometimes I yell, sometimes I cry when I'm angry. Do any of you do that?

Brittany: Mostly when I'm sad.

Therapist: Sometimes sadness mixes up with the anger.

MN: Brittany might be saying that for her; it would be easier for her to be sad than angry.

GD: At this moment, I wanted to concentrate on the complexity of anger as an emotion because that was really the prevailing emotion in the group at that time.

Melissa: When I'm really, really angry, I like to go in my room. I don't exactly slam the door. I do two things. I lock myself in my own closet and I scream for help or I go in my bed and jump and jump because I know my mom doesn't want me to.

MN: Interesting way to end the group: with provocation.

GD: It's fascinating how the letter elicited such different responses in this girls' group—concentrating on the mother–daughter dynamics, self-loathing, and discharge of anger in a range of ways.

MN: It shows how the letters elicit different responses in groups by gender and group constellation.

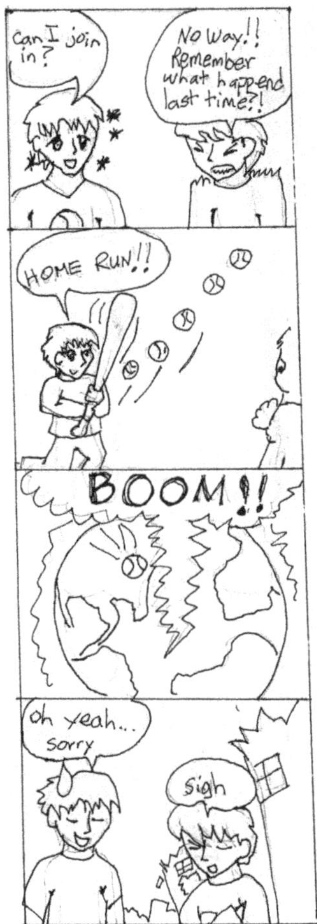
Can I join in?
No Way!! Remember what happend last time?!
HOME RUN!!
BOOM!!
oh yeah... sorry
sigh

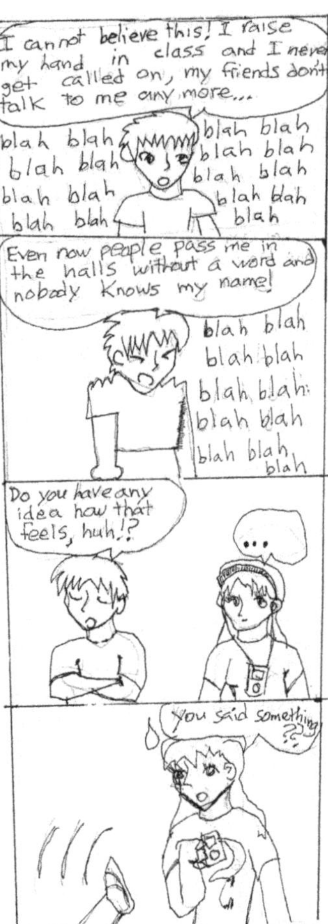
I can not believe this! I raise my hand in class and I never get called on, my friends don't talk to me any more...
blah blah blah blah blah blah blah blah blah blah blah blah blah blah blah
Even now people pass me in the halls without a word and nobody knows my name!
blah blah blah blah blah blah blah blah blah blah blah
Do you have any idea how that feels, huh!?
...
You said something ??

Suggested Activities

1. Place out a decorated cardboard box entitled "The Anger Box." Group members can decorate it with lightning bolts, red daggers, and so on. On a handout, ask each child to fill out the following and put their responses in the box. These can be read by the group leader to keep responses anonymous.
   a. I get angry every time____________.
   b. I blow up when ___________.
   c. When I lose my temper, I _____________.
   d. When I get angry and I do not want anyone to know it, I ______________.
   e. When someone is angry at me, I ____________________.
   f. A safe place to get angry is ___________________.
   g. When I get angry my face looks like ________ and my body looks like __________.
2. Circulate a sheet of packing bubble wrap. Each child tells something that makes them angry while they pop, twist, or mangle the bubble wrap.

References

Hall, K. (2001). *Asperger syndrome, the universe and everything*. London: Jessica Kingsley Publishers.

Klin, A., Volkmar, F. R., & Sparrow, S. S. (Eds.). (2000). *Asperger syndrome*. New York: Guilford Press.

Siegel, D. (1999). *The developing mind: How relationships and the brain interact to shape who we are*. New York: Guilford Press.

Winnicott, D. W. (1965). *The family and individual development*. London: Tavistock.

CHAPTER **11**

Behind Closed Doors

As school-aged children mature and approach pre-adolescence and adolescence, they test limits in new ways, often less conspicuously than younger children might do (Collins, 1995). In addition, the internet offers new temptations to children who may be intrigued and "inspired" to look at inappropriate websites. Some youngsters make secret purchases using their parents' credit cards. Often these "adventures" happen in the privacy of the child's own bedroom. This makes the mischievous deed even more compelling and exciting because the child perceives that he has gotten away with something. Secrecy clearly has a thrill about it. Such behaviors often go unchecked, until one day a parent discovers the child's computer history and learns what sites he's visited, or an interesting and unexpected package arrives at the front door. For children who struggle with impulse control, the immediate feedback they need is missing: the problematic behavior might go on for several weeks, or longer, until parents let their child know most emphatically that they have crossed the line. In dealing with these problems as they are manifested during these stages of development, it is important for parents to remember that there are two issues that drive all pre-adolescent and adolescent youngsters: (1) the need to save face and (2) the need to be in control. Getting caught is one way in which youngsters experience losing face. Being sneaky in order to get one's way, despite parental proscription, is a way of manifesting control (Collins & Laursen, 2004; Vgotsky, 1978). The following letter, and the group members' responses to it demonstrate this, among other issues.

Dear Kids' Club,

I have gotten myself in some serious trouble. We're talking major hot water! I love to go on the computer, Instant Message™ my friends, check out websites, and play computer games. I spend a couple of hours a day doing this. It's my biggest hobby. The other day I decided to get myself one of those neat CD players, so I ordered one on the internet using my mom's credit card. When my mom found out, she hit the ceiling. I told her I would do chores to pay for it, but that didn't seem to help. Then there is something else I did, too. I don't know how she found this out, but I went surfing on the net and found a porn site. I'm at that age where these things interest me, so I was just doing what other kids do. She is really mad now and has grounded me from my computer privileges for the next two weeks. I don't think the punishment fits the crime. She says that this is a "tip of the iceberg," that I am a big sneak and a liar. Next time I have to figure out a way to cover up better what I do on the computer. I am having a really hard time without having the computer to play with. I'm getting depressed about this and all I can do is to watch TV. So what is your advice?

Signed,
Chucky, the computer whiz kid
(Sarah, girl's version)

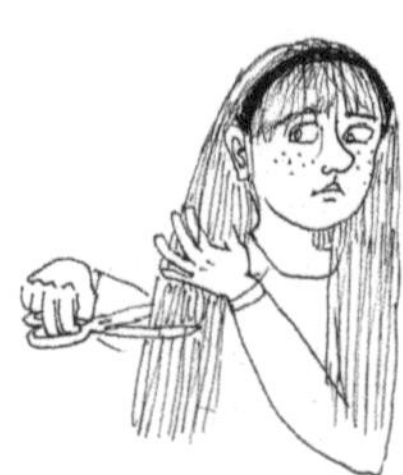

Boys' Group #2

Kevin: It was really wrong what you did, but I think that your mom is seriously over-reacting. I mean one time I accidentally went to a porn site. I was just surfing and somehow ....

MN: Somehow?

Kevin: ... I ended up on that site. My mom didn't take it too bad and she understood that. Your mom is seriously over-reacting. Did you try to go on to that?

MN: Listening to Kevin, we really don't know if he was trying to rationalize the boy's behavior or if he didn't understand what the letter-writer did.

Therapist: Yes, he did try to do this.

GD: I wanted to put the volition behind the action, so that Kevin really would understand what the boy had done.

Kevin: Then your mom is over-reacting, but it's not the end of the world. She doesn't need to ground you on the computer. You can also install a blocker.

MN: Although Kevin's responses were problematic, he kept the group speaking directly to the letter-writer. I like that. He stayed on-task, and kept the group on-task, irrespective of the quality of what he said.

GD: It's almost as if Kevin did not hear the letter accurately or that I pointed out again that he (the letter-writer) purposely did what he did. Kevin frequently did impulsive things, then reacted when others were upset with him, "I didn't do it! You're blaming me for nothing."

MN: That's a good example of the need to save face. Kevin also was saying that he needed external controls to stop him, because he lacked the internal ones. He required an auxiliary superego. There was an interaction of his dysregulated impulsivity with his moral development. It seems that his constitutionally based impulsive behavior caused him to get into the kind of trouble that he felt the need to justify instead of think about.

Julian: If you ask me, you shouldn't have done that. If you are intentionally doing that, then you deserve what you got. Actually I'd say that your mom is *under*-reacting. If you're going to that site on purpose, here's my advice if you're planning on doing that in the future. Don't!

MN: It's clear that the boys were attending to the pornography rather than the credit card misuse. It took the girls much longer to get to the porn.

Ian: Look, Chuck, once I went to a video game site and I saw all these anime pop-ups, so I quit on one and ended up on a porn one. Yeah. If you see it, just press X and get out of there. Forget all about it and say, "I'm done." And using your mom's credit card is not right at all. I mean, I have an iPod™, I think they cost a lot—like $500. If you think working-off chores can make that right, you'd have to work for eight or nine months to make that much. I think you're actually kind of lucky. If my mom caught me going on a website like that or using her credit card, she'd probably ground me for like a year and take the computer out of my room and only get to use it unless an adult is nearby. So, man, you're lucky.

MN: This was very pleasant and appealing to me. Ian had also touched on both of the important issues in the letter, something the group hadn't yet done. He was the first youngster able to do this. He implied that youngsters this age might have curiosity about these sites. That's one part. The other aspect is the outrage at the theft by credit card proxy, which is of course unacceptable. The $500 crossed the line for him. He came up with a responsible solution. "Get the computer out of the room." He suggested creating physical distance between himself and the temptations of the computer.

GD: Ian's parents were very involved and responsible parents who had worked hard to help him internalize right from wrong. Consequently, he was developing a high level of moral development and serving as an example to the group.

MN: He had internalized a sense of conscience. He understood that the losing of privileges and the need for extra controls hinges on the failure of trustworthiness.

Aidan: I have a suggestion for you. You are such a retard for going on that. You have some serious problems and you should cut it out.

GD: Aidan had done what the letter-writer had done. I changed some of the details in the letter to protect his privacy.

Aidan: If you're going on websites, that's one thing. If you're looking for porn, you've got to get advice and get some serious therapy. That's really wrong. Man, if you actually think about it, you're doing something that not many people do.

MN: If he only knew!

GD: Fortunately, he didn't yet.

Aidan: If you're actually looking for it, then you've got to get some help. And by using your mom's credit card, you're out of your mind. You could go in debt for that. You are so lucky that you're grounded for two weeks. If my mom caught me doing that, Oh my gosh! She would put off every privilege I have and make me earn it back. She would probably take out half the money in my bank account. She would ground me for about three years. Seriously. You got so lucky. Going on a porn site, using your mom's credit card, and saying, "I don't know how my mom found out." You're lucky she found out. You are so lucky.

GD: Aidan's impulse control went beyond his own difficulties in monitoring his own behavior. His father was an alcoholic who spent long hours on the computer gambling on sweepstakes, and sometimes looking at porn. It was possible that when Aidan went on the computer, pop-ups appeared. He had also probably observed his father doing these things.

MN: The language he used suggests how different he was from Ian. Ian had internalized external controls whereas Aidan's tone was angry and unraveled. The group's process is actually using the letter-writer's material as a way of talking about issues of moral development.

Julian: Also, with the credit card thing. By the way, could I ask you a question? Are you insane? Because, look, Aidan's right. If your mom hadn't found out until later, you could end up homeless.

MN: That was rather a Draconian statement. Did Julian have that strict a superego? Or was he more concerned, on a lower level of moral development, with the punishment he might receive?

GD: I think that Julian needed rules delineated in black and white terms. He often struggled when a situation required more sophisticated reasoning and judgment. He was a brilliant child who lacked the ability to read social cues. He also depended on factual rules and guidelines to learn how to live his life.

Julian: Actually I'm surprised that your mom didn't ground you for life. That's what you deserve!

MN: Julian's intensity of outrage is interesting; he was so involved in this. I wonder why?

GD: Julian didn't anticipate things that could have happened, and then he was surprised when he found himself in difficult situations. Frequently he was ostracized by boys at school and teased without mercy because of the things he did. Unfortunately, he had no awareness that his own behaviors triggered those responses in others. He was very intelligent but lacked social awareness. In looking at the group process, notice that I hadn't needed to speak for quite a while. The kids were grabbing the microphone from one another. The energy in the room was quite charged.

MN: You didn't need to clarify issues or validate them. In a positive sense, the therapist was irrelevant during this segment of the session. The group didn't need the therapist to say anything because the kids were running the process by themselves. In a way, it's what we want: to shift from being group leaders to being group facilitators and commentators.

GD: It showed the maturity of the group, at least of the boys when they were in the group.

Ian: I just want to have one last comment. Stay away, the computer is evil!

Aidan: There's one other thing. Your mom should be a little more updated and she should have some kind of porn blocker. If you didn't have that, something else could happen. Ask your mom to get a blocker.

GD: I told Aidan's mother to get a blocker immediately and protect all the computers in the house. Aidan was on his father's computer when he got into trouble. Aidan knew that I was involved in this process.

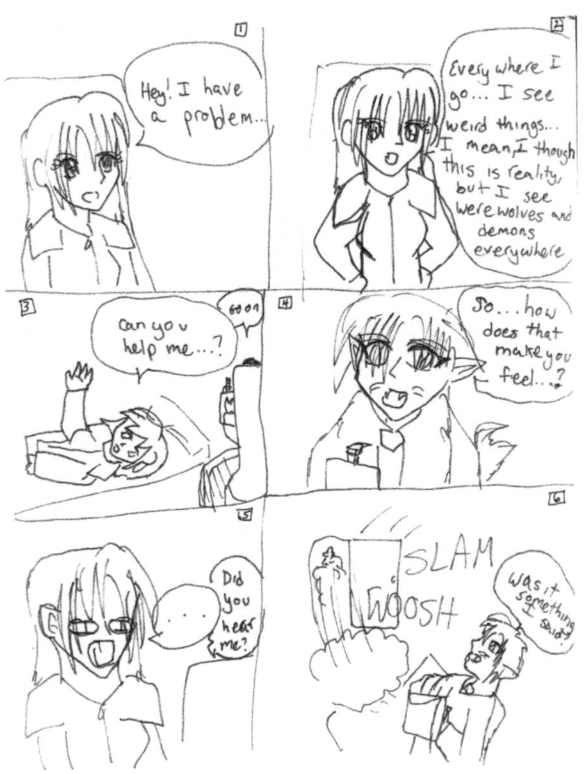
1
Hey! I have a problem...
2
Every where I go... I see weird things... I mean, I though this is reality, but I see werewolves and demons everywhere
3
can you help me...?
Go on
4
So... how does that make you feel...?
5
...
Did you hear me?
6
SLAM
WOOSH
Was it something I said?

Boys' Group #3

GD: At the end of last week's group, Leo wrote the following letter and handed it to me. He wanted me to read it to the group. We included it in this book to give an example of the kind of letter that children in the groups began to write, wanting advice from their own groups.

MN: So the groups were developing to the point where they could, at least some of the time, create their own "stimulus narratives," rather than rely on the letters that you had generated.

> *Yo boys' club:*
>
> I have a serious anger management problem. A kid on the other team called our team "sucky" and I kicked him in the shins. He was OK and I didn't get suspended. I really need some advice. How would you help me? Help me, guys, especially Justin, please.
>
> **Signed,**
> **Anonymouse**

Justin: Why me? He must have heard that I'm an expert on anger management.

GD: It's hilarious that Leo didn't think that by naming Justin he blew his anonymous cover. The boys didn't know that this letter came from one of them. Leo asked me to introduce the letter as if it were from a boy from another boys' group.

Corey: If you have an anger management problem, then you should go to a therapist. Try not to hit or kick or touch anybody. You should try to calm yourself down. Ask your parents or your coach to help you. Whatever you do, don't throw a beer.

Oliver: My advice to you, anonymouse, whoever you are, you should try not to get annoyed by Mitchell doing his stupid victory dance whenever he scores a goal.

Nate: Ummmmm (knocking on the mike).

Therapist: I'll bet every guy in here has had an anger blow up. Think of a time that you had that happen to you and what helped you.

Nate: Find a friend and that will help you.

Jamie: First thing about this stupid victory dance and when he calls your team "sucky," tell on him or hire somebody to do it for you to beat him up.

MN: That was a bit off, hiring a hit man! A bit of Mafioso posturing. Even though Jamie might be kidding, he was nevertheless demonstrating the morally immature illusion that having someone else do the dirty deed would somehow absolve him of responsibility.

Justin: First of all be careful if you hear Leo talking. Be prepared for no good answers. I have had a lot of anger first hand. You should set up an APS-Anger Prevention Strategies! Like you should find ways like my APS. Like in my APS, I do reading because reading calms me down. Or body pressure. See if you can get therapists to apply pressure to your body if it's available. You should also talk to an adult, like your coach. Think before you act and I say, so long.

MN: Leo was right to ask Justin.

GD: And Justin came through for him. That's Justin. During this discussion, Leo had a great deal of difficulty focusing on the discussion. He was very agitated that we were talking about his problem and was goofing around, looking at his book, and not paying attention to the discussion. I transcribed it for him and gave him Justin's advice in an outline form. He was emotionally flooded because his letter was being talked about.

MN: Did he really want you to read it to the group?

GD: Yes, he did. I think he was trying to act as if it wasn't his letter.

MN: That's the need to save face.

GD: This letter is a wonderful example of the process that the Kids' Club letters might ignite in group psychotherapy.

Suggested Activities

1. Make a "Dummy's Guide to Anger Management" instructional videotape using material generated from last week's anger box. Focus on ways of "putting on the brakes" or on safe ways to express anger and how to think before acting. The group leader can "freeze the action," then ask a child to say what she is thinking or feeling at that moment. The leader can hold a thought bubble or a heart-shaped piece of

paper over the child's head to depict "What is she thinking or feeling?" Then resume action to continue the story line.

2. Using clay or a similar medium, make individual or a group sculpture. While working the clay, talk with the children about how this is a way to help channel angry feelings by using resistive mediums and making something that might depict how they feel inside.

References

Collins, W. A. (1995). Relationships and development: Family adaptation to individual change. In S. Shulman (Ed.), *Close relationships and socioemotional development* (pp. 128–154). New York: Ablex.

Collins, W. A., & Laursen, B. (2004). Family relationships and parenting influences. In R. Lerner, & L. Steinberg (Eds.), *Handbook of adolescent psychology* (pp. 331–362). New York: Wiley.

Vgotsky, L. (1978). *Mind and society*. Cambridge, MA: Harvard University Press.

CHAPTER 12
Who's the Boss? "I'm the Boss!"

All children need to learn how to share control with others. The inhibited-and-anxious child, just as he feels at the mercy of his feelings, may well experience a lack of control in his life in general, allowing others to boss him around. Others make decisions for him, and, due to poorly developed autonomy this may comfort the anxious child. However, this pattern leads the child eventually to feel even more inadequate and socially incompetent (Brooks & Siegel, 1996; Greenspan, 2003). In contrast, the more oppositional child seeks the role of boss/foreman and is unable to share control with others. Behavioral inflexibility pervades day-to-day interactions and everyday routines, and children with this attribute have difficulty trying something new and prefer things to be done exactly and predictably the same way each time. By assuming total control, they attempt to ensure their own sovereignty over predictability. These children may appear to be oppositionally defiant for its own sake, when in fact they are desperate for the maintenance of sameness in their environment for constitutional reasons (Barkley & Benton, 1998).

One example of anxiety-based need for control, as well as behavioral inflexibility, can be observed in a child who becomes increasingly rigid about events and objects. He might not want others to touch his playthings; he may wish for everything to be done a certain way each time; and he may not be able to tolerate the slightest deviation in rules. One often sees a child like this who needs the game to be played by his own set of rules or conversely he may require rigid adherence to the game's actual rules. When this doesn't happen according to plan, such children tend to blow up, become disruptive, or summarily end the game for all concerned. Clearly, we can expect these children to have a hard time with everyday routines and not to allow parents to steer them to the next activity within expected time frames (Gillot, Furniss, & Walter, 2001).

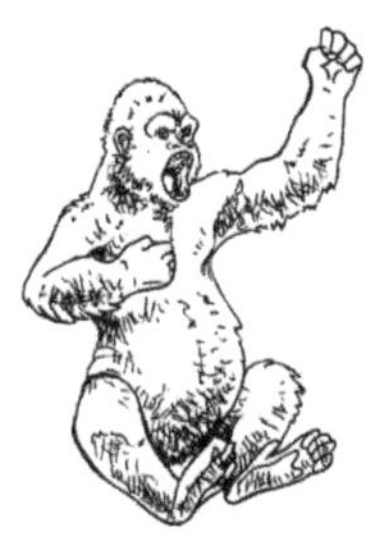

Dear Kids' Club,

I am a finicky kind of kid. I don't like people telling me what to do and how to do it. I get in my mind the way I want things to go and that's the way I want it. It's like I have a set of directions in my head and once the reel starts, I have to keep going with the script. This could be a good trait, but unfortunately I get into a lot of fights when I have a friend over. I don't want him touching my stuff and I want to pick the game and do things my way. The other day, Tommy was over and he started opening up my closet and looking at my collections, moving the things around and messing it all up. I exploded and told him to "Get out of my house, NOW!" He probably won't come over again after that.

I also like to follow the rules in games. I hate it when kids make up their own rules or do things different from what the game rules are supposed to be. I freaked out recently in a game of Cadoo™ when the kids did the game different than it says in the game book. There's a vein in my neck that literally pops out when I get that mad.

The long and short of this is that I like to be in charge and to be the boss of situations. As long as I have control, am picked to be the leader, can pick the games we play, I'm good. If someone else is the leader, I can feel my stomach start jumping around inside. I usually try to get to be the one in charge and sometimes I'm pretty clever about maneuvering that. If I can't do what I want or have planned, then I blow up, storm out of the room, or pick a fight with the boss kid. I usually bring my playing cards to the playground and if I can set up a game, I'm in heaven. The other day the kids said they were sick of playing cards with me. When they insisted on playing Capture the Flag, I took one of my cards and hurled it at Nick's forehead. He deserved what he got because he was so pushy about it and insulting to me and my interests.

Anyway, what do you think about all this?

Signed,
Rick, the Rigid Guy
(Rita in girl's version)

MN: There are two possibilities that may be helpful in understanding this "phantom youngster." One is to take his comments strictly at face value: that he is simply a controlling, bullying sort of child. The other possibility is that he is a child with a regulatory issue who is trying to take control because he can't deal with unexpected things or non-predictable outside stimulation in general. He feels like a perpetually potential dartboard. In order for him to feel regulated, he has to be extremely controlling. Another possibility is that this is a child with both control issues and a regulatory problem. Thus, the bullying behavior is socially maladaptive, but functionally adaptive if we understand the self-regulation contributor to his problem.

GD: This is not simply a child with obsessive-compulsive disorder who has inflexibility and rigidity in his personality. The child in this letter, actually, is based on many of the children I have seen who experience a combination of regulatory issues that derail their capacity to tolerate change. I also tried to put into the letter some of the bodily sensations that these children sometimes experience, such as their stomachs jumping around. The body is not well regulated and this contributes to the child's emotional dysregulation.

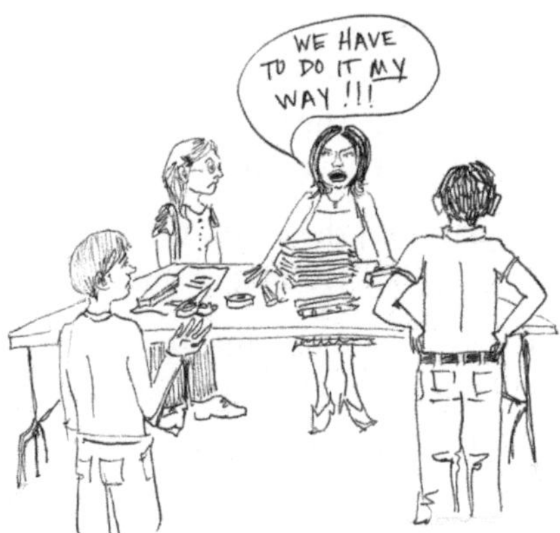

Girls' Group #2

Annie: If you are who I think you are, when you do that when I come over, I don't want to stay.

GD: She really thinks this is a person she knows.

MN: It would be interesting to see if she would say this as directly if she thought it were someone who happened to be in the group. Then the issue of confrontation would be raised, and there would be a dual opportunity for the therapist and therefore for the group. Direct confrontation of a specific person could lead to the confronter gaining a better understanding of her impact on other people. This is one of the goals of group therapy: learning how we impact others. In addition, the group itself could learn more effective ways of confronting one another.

GD: It wasn't any other group member. It's really a shame because it didn't give us the opportunity to deal with these things. I'm sometimes frustrated by how the group process just doesn't allow us to follow some issues that we know could be helpful. We can only do so much in any one session.

Annie: I really, really don't like it. You should try to let somebody else pick the game.

MN: She was trying to teach the social effect on others to help the writer understand her effect on other kids. This was helpful. As the opening group statement, a therapist would hope to be able to keep this issue alive throughout the session.

GD: It just occurred to me who she thinks this is. Annie was friendly with a girl who was in another one of my groups. This letter is not about that girl at all.

Briana: If I came over, I'd probably think so too. I'd want to get out of your house. You should try letting them look and see what they do with it. Like if they're taking stuff down and throwing it on the floor, then tell them to stop and that you don't like it. But until then, let them see stuff. They may compliment you on it. Try some new games and you might like that person as a leader. It may be more fun and you've never tried it before and you might find it fun.

GD: Briana used to be very similar to Rita, the girl in the letter, with a high need to control others.

MN: I believe that Briana was saying that you should wait and see, not make assumptions, and give others a chance. Don't just write them off. We can see through this comment how, and what, she was learning from being in group.

GD: Yes, I don't think this would have happened without the group.

Chelsea: If you don't want to play with the cards, try to make card castles. It's hard to do. Try playing Capture the Flag. It's a lot of fun.

MN: Again we've seen Chelsea's resourcefulness. She was saying that if a bossy child whom you're visiting is trying to impose a game on you, change it into something that works for the two of you. It is a hard thing to do.

GD: What she was saying sounds simple and her language was like a child her age, but her solution was, in a way, sophisticated.

MN: I agree. She was actually working with diplomacy.

Ellen: You can try to find a girl who likes to do things with you, someone who doesn't want to be a leader who would like someone to show them their things.

Annie: If you are who I think you are, I don't think what Ellen said is a good idea. I don't really like being the leader, but I still don't like it when you do that stuff.

MN: Ellen was saying that the bully should find someone she can have influence over without having to resort to bullying, find someone who wants to be led. She was trying to create a transformation from aggression to assertion. I suspect that she was also picking up the bully's underlying sense of feeling at the mercy of others. The bully has to become the controller because otherwise she will feel victimized by others. This was all being said in implicit communication. Annie, on the other hand, said that being led by someone else would not be a satisfactory solution for her. It is fascinating to see two youngsters of similar temperament attempt to deal with a bully in such different ways. Ellen's comment was hinted at some empathy for the bully, while Annie responded to her own feelings. This presents the therapist with a choice point in facilitating the group.

GD: Yes. Do you choose to help the group understand a bully so that they can find solutions for themselves by using that understanding, or do you work instead with what it feels like to be bullied? In this case, the group decided for itself: continue with advice for the bully. By themselves, they chose the "helpfulness route" and I think this came from some ability, on a group level, to try to empathize with—not approve of—the girl in the letter.

Briana: What you should do is instead of having her come over and want to do something, you can set up what you want to play with her and let her choose. Tell her that the rest of the games that aren't set up are not for playing with that day. Or you can make a list of things to play with and do it in order or have her pick from the list.

Maya: You could let her choose the first thing to play and let her be the leader, then you can choose the next game and you can be the leader.

MN: This was nice advice but I don't know if the letter-writer could have used these strategies. The group members are not actually commenting on each other's suggestions. They are primarily speaking to the letter-writer. Dynamically, then, the letter-writer became the leader of the group.

GD: It's true that the girls weren't talking to each other, but they ***were*** listening to each other. They were bringing themselves to the advice they were giving. I decided not to pick up on this group process style but instead to let them give their advice. That's because they were attuned to the content of the letter and I thought aspects of the letter's issue were touching them.

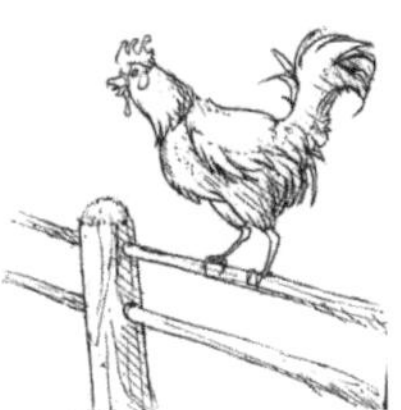

Boys' Group #1

Duncan: Hello, Rick. I would say, just keep doing what you're doing. If you're the boss, the hell with them.

MN: Duncan was presenting both a clinical question and a technical issue for the therapist. Clinically, he may have simply seemed identified with the bully and therefore had a degree of ego-syntonic aggression toward others. On the other hand, he may have been identifying with the aggressor because he unconsciously experienced himself as personally victimized. Perhaps literally victimized by others, or internally victimized in the sense of being at the mercy of his own feelings.

GD: There was a decision to be made by the therapist. Duncan's comment was the opening comment in the group.

MN: Does the therapist permit this line of response even though it truly goes against the intent of the session? Or does the therapist see Duncan's response as a potential derailment of the group and therefore bring the group back to the letter and thus to the true issue?

GD: I decided to bring the group back. I thought that Duncan's comment could have become a group-level diversion. I didn't want that to happen, at least not from a single comment by one group member at the beginning of the session.

Therapist: Well, that's why he's writing. He's having a problem. He's getting into hot water because of this problem. It's not working. He likes being the boss and everyone's getting angry at him about it. He's stuck in wanting to be in control. He wants to know how not to always be in control, and tolerate it because it is his nature.

Javier: I don't know how to help you with the problem. I'm just saying, frankly, that if you're not in control, you exploding isn't going to hurt anybody but yourself, unless you chuck something at someone. Then you'll be in even deeper hot water. The other person is going to be yelling at you, too.

GD: Whenever I used my larger therapy room for the group, Javier went through my cabinets, drawers, all my closets, and rooted around my things without permission. He became completely dysregulated in a larger, more stimulating environment. He also became rigid and controlling when he couldn't anticipate and plan for events in his life. I'm interested that he said here, "I don't know how to help you with the problem." He was overwhelmed.

MN: He was aware that there is a limit to socially unacceptable behavior; there are interpersonal consequences. Then he got stuck and really didn't know what to do.

Therapist: Do you have any suggestions for what he can do when he's getting angry when he can't be in control?

Javier: If you're going to blow up, my advice is to leave the room so that you don't chuck something at someone. And wait to cool down. If you can't do that, stay out of the room until you have cooled down.

GD: That is the strategy that I had coached Javier to use—to leave the room, collect himself, and then return to the group in a productive way. Whenever he got angry in the group, I coached him to walk the balance beam 10 times out in the hallway and then return.

Jacob: What you could do is pretend to play along with him, then mess up the whole game. Then you play your game and hope that nobody messes it up.

MN: Sweet revenge! No group member responded to that. That's a bit surprising. Why do you think that is?

GD: Because Jacob was so annoying. He purposely maneuvered and manipulated things in the group to get his way. The kids couldn't stand him, so I think they backed off. They didn't want to be bothered with him.

MN: So the group was experiencing a reenactment of what the letter-writer was saying. There it was, right in front of you. Jacob was the bully and the other boys didn't want anything to do with him. It would have been wonderful if someone in the group, some brave soul, had drawn the similarity between Jacob and the letter-writer.

GD: Yes. They were all backing away from him. It was absolutely a parallel process.

Therapist: Everybody likes to be in control sometimes. I'm a girl and I like to cook. When I have friends over, sometimes I don't like them interfering with me, like grabbing bowls and throwing things in. I like to be in charge of my own kitchen. It gets me a little rattled when I see people just barge in and take over my kitchen. I was wondering if any of you have anything you really want to be in charge of and you don't like someone messing in it?

GD: I thought perhaps that it might be helpful to normalize the need for control with a personal example.

Tyrone: Sometimes at school if we're playing a game and we're working on a project, if no one is working on the project, I hate telling everyone to try to get the work done. I don't know if they're going to yell at me.

MN: I think Tyrone was trying to say that he's not naturally a bully, and that when there was a situation in which he wanted or needed to take control, it troubled him. He didn't want to alienate anyone. He was picking up the alienation and helplessness that the letter-writer felt. He may also have been frightened of his own aggressive fantasies.

GD: Rather than express this, Tyrone attended to the social implications of being a bully. From a group process framework; it was a good solution. He was pursuing an important issue while protecting himself from the anxiety that had been evoked by the aggression in the letter.

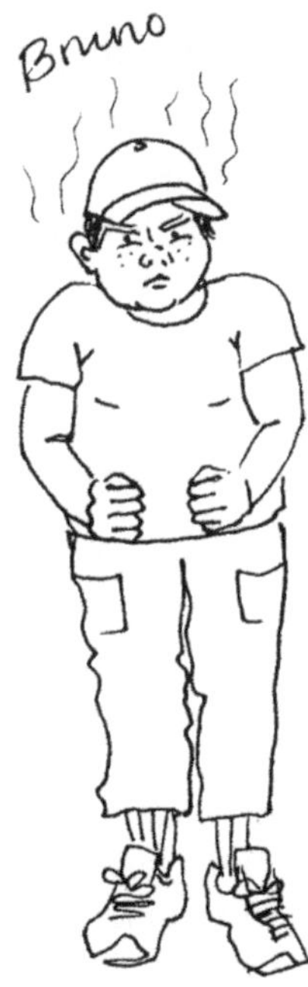

Therapist: That's a different kind of problem about being a leader. You might be unpopular if you take the lead.

Javier: Actually my problem is almost the exact opposite of yours. In a school project, this used to happen a lot, particularly in social studies, which I loved. We would always be getting a project to learn history. It worked, it really did. The group was planning something and they'd all be talking. Usually what would happen is that everyone would have a different plan and everyone would be talking at once. They'd all be trying to work out this plan. Even if I had a suggestion that I thought would be good and probably would have made the group quicker or more efficient, I could not stand being in that crowd of four different desks. The noise and the closeness. I couldn't get a word in edgewise and I couldn't stand it.

MN: That seems clearly to be a regulatory or processing problem.

GD: Yes, it is. Whenever there was a group team project like building something, Javier cleared the room, grabbed all the pieces, and had to be in complete control of the entire project. If someone else touched even one piece or had a different idea, he would protest. I think he struggled with processing other people's ideas and integrating them into his own, in addition to being overwhelmed on a sensory level by the noise, movement, and random physical touching by peers.

Therapist: I'm glad you brought this up because I think that that's part of Rick's problem.

MN: This is an example of functional group process. Javier was able to continue and the group remained non-disruptive.

Javier: So I would just hover around the edges until they solidified their plan. The main problem there is that is I got stuck with a job I didn't like. I couldn't do anything much about it. I could protest, but then we'd have to start all over again.

Therapist: Thanks for bringing that up, Javier. I think that you're hitting the nail on the head about something that Rick hasn't really thought about yet.

MN: This is an example of how positive group dynamics proceed. Duncan picked up the theme.

Duncan: Well, when I'm playing my Star Wars™ (video) game or building something, sometimes my Mom or my sister will try to come by and help, and it's like "HELLO! I'm doing this on my own; I don't need your help. Thank you very much. Now leave me alone." But it's mostly with the Star Wars™ game. When I'm on the game, I think, "There! I finally finished this and now I can start something new on the game."

Therapist: So you prefer working alone?

Duncan: Mostly on projects, I prefer individual projects instead of group.

MN: Duncan experienced others who were working with him or trying to help him on a project as if they were intrusive bullies who wanted to take over. He tried to get in control in a reactive way. "Get out of my way. Leave me alone. This is what I am doing. Stop it!" This was different from the letter-writer.

GD: It was a different form of isolation. He regressed into isolation which seemed both a processing problem of integrating multiple inputs at once, as well as an emotional need to be alone and avoid interactions with others. Duncan needed to plan all the steps without interruption. It was obviously difficult for Duncan to work in groups and this had implications for his school functioning.

Suggested Activities

1. Create two teams and have children answer questions from the Talking, Feeling, and Doing Game™. Instead of using the game board, the group leader asks the questions from the game cards, one card per team, rotating who gets to answer the question. Points can be awarded to the teams for their answers.
2. If the children need something more active, play the Survivor Challenge™ game.

References

Barkley, R. A., & Benton, C. M. (1998). *Your defiant child.* New York: Guilford Press.

Brooks, B., & Siegel, P. M. (1996). *The scared child: Helping kids overcome traumatic events.* New York: Wiley.

Greenspan, S. I. (2003). *The secure child: Helping children feel safe and confident in a changing world.* Cambridge, MA: DeCapo.

Gillot, A., Furniss, F., & Walter, A. (2001). Anxiety in high functioning children with autism. *Autism*, 5, 277–286.

CHAPTER 13
Alone on a Desert Island

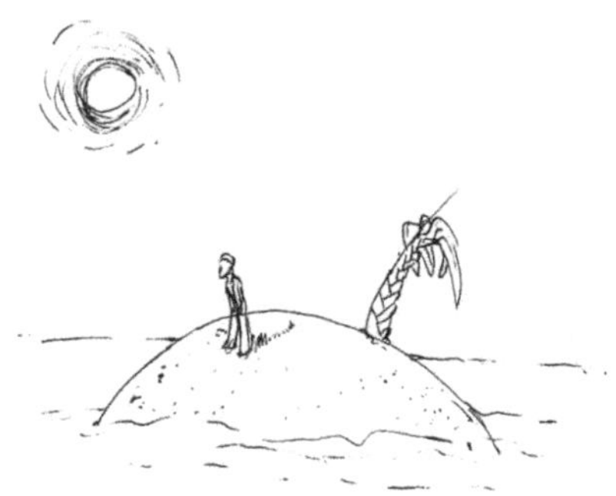

Shy and withdrawn behavior occurs in childhood for many reasons. Some children are born temperamentally slow-to-warm to others and may struggle all their lives with the difficulties of social approach (Carey & McDevitt, 1995; Greenspan & Salmon, 1996). Practice sometimes helps these youngsters learn how to make social overtures. Other children remain so anxious that they become phobic about social interchanges (Brooks & Siegel, 1996).

Peers often ignore the shy, withdrawn, child. This reinforces a "cycle of isolation." Some children are outwardly rejected by peers for their social awkwardness. Usually a shy child develops social passivity and never masters ways to be assertive. However, some of these children become oppositional at home. This is their way of trying to find avenues for self-assertion and control. Learning to balance appropriate control whether at home or in the social arena is often a clearly difficult developmental task (DeGangi & Kendall, 2008).

As children enter school, the outward social rejection often becomes internalized. Thus, they may take on themselves the rejection they have experienced from other youngsters. Such children, feeling painfully excluded by peers, develop patterns of isolation. One feature of internalization is the development of depression, often the result of the child's perception of being unlikable to peers. The problem becomes exacerbated when a child is also physically clumsy and struggles to participate in sports activities. This youngster may be teased for a speech impediment or for running in an awkward fashion. In addition, many children with constitutional problems have food allergies that set them apart socially. Imagine the child with a peanut allergy who has to eat at a separate table at school. Finally, some children who are shy and withdrawn simply have no idea how to converse in natural conversations with peers (Klass & Costello, 2003).

Dear Kids' Club,

It is really hard for me to write this letter. I am really shy and have a hard time thinking of what to say or do with other kids. I'm what you call "slow-to-warm-up." When kids are playing, I usually go off by myself and find something to do by myself. Recently I have gotten in the habit of bringing a book along to read because I get left out so much. At lunch I eat by myself at the food allergy table because of my peanut allergies. Right now there is only one other kid who eats there and he sits at the other end of the table.

Am I happy about being so shy? I don't think so, but maybe this is how things are going to be for me the rest of my life. I don't have any friends except my cousins who are older than me. They like to show me how to do different computer games and one of them likes to read the same kind of books I read.

I guess the part of this that does bother me is that kids tease me about the way I talk and what I wear. They call me "The Mumbler" because I talk under my breathe in a soft voice whenever I have something to say, which isn't much to start with. I just look away or down at my shoes when they say, "Hey, here's the Mumbler!" There are some other kids who ask me why I still wear stretchy pants, white socks, and my favorite t-shirt every day. It's what I like to wear. They say that I'm a big dweeb. They poke at my stomach when they say that to me. It's really embarrassing. I just try to stay to myself and keep away from everyone.

Do you have any advice for me?

Signed,
Mike the Mumbler (and Dweeb)
(Michele in girls' version)

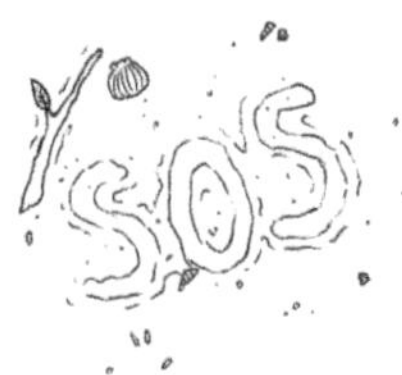

Girls' Group #2

Annie: I used to not have any friends and all I could do at recess was walk. Then I told this person who is my friend that I didn't have any friends and she let me be her friend. You just have to find somebody who is really nice. When I get to know someone, I talk different. This is how I talk in school. (She is talking in a very soft voice), "Ahhh . . . mumble . . . ."

MN: We can hear, in this statement, Annie's sad urgency to be understood. I think that's why she demonstrated the problem with her softly voiced re-enactment. If she hadn't done this "demonstration" of herself, it wouldn't have had the same immediacy. She wanted the other group members, and you, to know that the letter was speaking to her and that she was in pain. Thus, the group began with an expression of heartfelt sadness and claiming of the problem.

GD: She even said "Ahhh . . . mumble," the same words from the letter, expressing a very strong identification with the letter-writer. This had the potential to really "grab" the group right from the start.

MN: She was not only describing her problem; she was being it, in the moment.

Therapist: You do that at school? (She replied, "Yes"). It's so different how you are here. Do any other girls have advice for Michele?

GD: I returned to the letter-writer because I was responding to a certain feeling in the group. I felt that it was too painful for the group to focus on Annie—a person in the room whose problem was so close to the letter-writer's. Usually Annie would be rather agitated and tip her chair back and forth through the entire session. At that moment she was crumpled over in half while talking. I wanted to protect her by backing away. I hoped to return later to how she was feeling, after she had emotionally restored herself enough to receive our feedback and help.

Latisha: Maybe find someone with the same interests or someone who doesn't have a friend so that they would be really happy to have you as a friend. Try ignoring the people who tease you.

Ellen: I don't know exactly what I do because I'm shy. You can go and play with them, and they won't stop you from playing with them. I have a speech impediment and get speech therapy for it.

MN: Ellen's juxtaposition of these two comments: (1) "You can go and play with them, and they won't stop you from playing with them," and (2) "I have a speech impediment and get speech therapy" was important. She was talking about something that's wrong with her. I don't really know if she was also making a comment about her difficulty with friends. It's almost an example of magical thinking. "You can go and play with them and they won't stop you from playing with them." This needs translation. This often happens in therapy. Comments can often be taken at face value and then suddenly we may get something that is a metaphor and therefore a shift in the group language.

GD: I had the same thought. Ellen's obstacle was emotional but the speech impediment was nested on top of it. She perceived her speech problem as the reason it was so hard for her to join with friends. She could make beautiful and insightful comments, but she usually held back because of her fear that her peers would make fun of her speech impediment.

Therapist: Ellen, do kids call you a name because of the way you speak?

Ellen: No.

Therapist: I understand you completely.

GD: I was referring to her speech with this comment. I wanted to affirm that there was nothing noticeably wrong. Most people would not have been able to hear any dysfluency.

Briana: There are a lot of reasons why you still do this. One is because you're not used to making big speeches. Number Two—you need to find somebody else who is just like you. Number Three—I think you need to start speaking more. Have a speech in front of your parents and practice. That will help you with your speaking up. If you want to ever be someone who is really important, you're going to have to make a lot of speeches. You need to practice. Talk to your teacher about that. She can help you. I'll bet you'll be making some speeches in school some time and you can get ready for that. My last piece of advice is in making friends, what you need to do is pray to God that you will find someone who is just like you. You'll probably get that person when you least expect it.

MN: The letter conveys a feeling of isolation that the girls were having trouble tolerating. They perceived the letter-writer as a child who was so shy that she couldn't do anything and so, defensively, they made recommendations like "Find somebody else who is just like you." But this child (the letter-writer) couldn't talk to anybody. How in the world was she going to "find someone just like you?" Dynamically, the group was using defensive denial of what the letter-writer's problem is: they took it away. They touched fleetingly on the isolation, but they were fixing it in a magical way that clearly was not realistic. A shy person is not going to run around to find somebody just like her. If she finds another shy person, she is not going to talk in response. "You need to speak up more and practice speeches in front of your parents" was Briana's recommendation. I think she became more concerned, at this moment, with making a good impression rather than on the emotional content.

GD: That was what Briana was all about—making impressions on others. She was very conscious about her appearance, her hair, her dress, and her pretty face, rather than the actual person she was. However, I was impressed by the leap she made, changing a shy, mumbling child and turning her into a speech-making President of the United States.

MN: The grandiosity of this shift makes me wonder if she was using reaction formation, protecting herself from feeling socially different and not worthwhile. That may be why clothes and makeup had an exaggerated importance. The isolation of the letter-writer touched her. And the "pray to God" comment seemed to reflect a sad need to turn to an all-powerful Someone to help her because she felt so helpless herself.

GD: Briana was very aware of all the special services she needed over the years, including occupational therapy, psychotherapy, and group therapy. She had to practice many skills to become successful socially. I think that she perceived herself as having a "failed body," a body that had basic things wrong with it.

Danielle: At my old school I used to be alone and I always brought a book out, then the teacher said "No" to me. During the end of the school year, I met this group of girls who I never knew before. They act like my friends and they all love to sing and dance and I became friends with them. Try to find a friend who you might like. Give speeches like you're on stage. If you're in a neighborhood, go up to kids and try to get play dates with them. The other girl at your allergy table, if she's not really mean to you, try talking to her. See if she has anything in common with you. Try sitting next to her in the next few weeks and see if she's nice.

GD: I was very pleased that Danielle chose to speak at this moment. Her face was usually buried in her book, a tiny child with dysmorphic features (e.g., unusual proportions and facial features) who looked three years younger than her age. She chose this moment in the course of the session to speak to the human need to attempt to reach out to others.

MN: She talked about how she used to bring a book out, yet she continued to sit in her current group with a book out. Giving speeches as if you are onstage is not a relationship. Briana did the same thing: picturing an "as-if" relationship, while actually putting distance between herself and anybody else. You can't make friends by standing on a stage and giving speeches because you're not talking to anybody in particular. This approach suggests the helplessness that the group was experiencing in figuring out how to connect with others. The group was reflecting the same "pray to God" feeling that Briana had expressed.

GD: Hopelessness was the pervasive group emotion. Both of these girls did not understand how to make interpersonal connections at all. They were both very challenged by the task of establishing intimacy and attachments with others. They were good representatives of the overall group feeling.

Maya: If people are playing games at recess, then you can go up to them and ask if you can play. See if there's a girl one day at recess and ask to play with her.

Latisha: I think that the girl at your allergy table, start a conversation and maybe she'll start one too.

Briana: Maybe you have something in common with somebody else and you can talk about that.

MN: Although they sound somewhat different, each of these girls was saying something that connected with what the other had said. Therefore, group-level communication was occurring even though it may not have appeared so on the surface. Group process took primacy over content here. As therapists, we always have to be ready to identify whether the process or the content is primary and therefore most healing. The balance shifts often, even within minutes, in each session.

GD: They were building a conversation on what the other had said. They were suggesting that they might need to be the ones who initiate an interaction to get things started in a friendship. Actually, they were practicing, through the group process, exactly what they were recommending to the letter-writer. This could not have happened in individual therapy.

Annie: I used to feel like a speck on the wall. Nobody noticed me or cared about me. I still feel that way sometimes. When I am very shy, everyone is always asking me, "What's wrong?" I hate that! I know exactly how Michele feels.

GD: That broke my heart!

MN: It was very poignant, and part of what is sad is that she was missing the opportunity. She felt "like a speck on the wall" when she was feeling shy. Yet when people came up to her and asked, "What's wrong?" she hated it. Given this statement, I think Annie's shyness was serving some defensive function for her—an avoidance of interactions.

GD: She was definitely rejecting the overtures of others. Annie used to fall deeper and deeper into her depressive hole and became that speck on the wall right before our eyes. She was a soulful child who often wrote moving poetry. Her talent was stunning and masterful. She could find her voice in her poems but couldn't find that voice with people.

MN: Did you worry what might happen to her when she became a late adolescent or an adult? You mentioned her poetry, and we have this example of her rejecting help. Is she a future Sylvia Plath or Anne Sexton—both of whom killed themselves?

GD: Annie had severe seasonal affective disorder and every winter she became quite depressed. A lot of her poetry was rather dark. I worried a lot about her future and hoped that the therapies, developing friendships, and family support would make a difference.

Danielle: If you have a pet or your favorite stuffed animals, try talking to them. That's what I usually do. They make you feel happier. Stuffed animals usually act like friends.

GD: She needed to shift to inanimate objects—things that couldn't talk to her.

MN: The group had moved to a safe place; they all talked about how they placed themselves at a distance from others. The therapist was at another choice point: what to follow through on. They were claiming their shyness. One choice might have been for the therapist to inquire—"Have you ever followed your own advice?" Another choice might have been to follow up on the shyness itself. And yet another one, one we sometimes forget, could be to stay silent and see where it goes.

GD: I think that the girls had decided that they were finished giving advice. The topic was upsetting them. The thought of being that isolated and owning these feelings was overwhelming. I chose silence and let the session end.

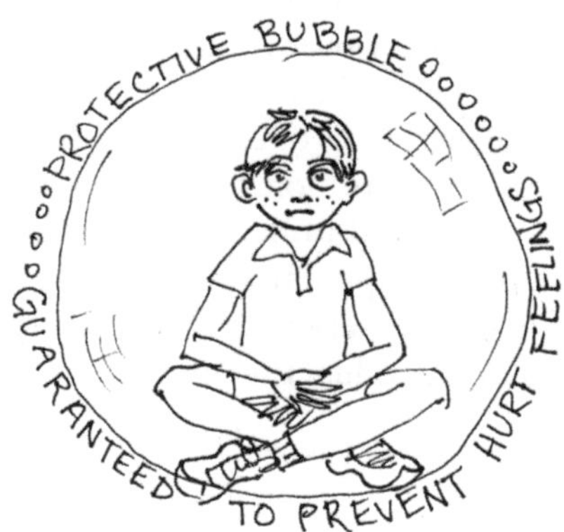

Boys' Group #3

Justin: I just wanted to say that you shouldn't be bothered if they call you dweeb or whatever. They're probably not so nice anyway. You probably will make some friends. I like to read by myself sometimes. So you know what, I have times when I just want to be alone. Just ignore those that don't treat you with respect. Try to make friends with those who would.

Jamie: Since you like books, you should really get into *Calvin and Hobbes* and you might make some friends that way. You could try playing freeze tag once in a while.

MN: Jamie was referring to finding a common interest. Youngsters are into the *Calvin and Hobbes* comic strip books. It's turning around what Justin said—using books to be alone. Jamie was using the comic books to join others. He was saying, "Look for the commonalities between you and other kids." It's easier when you have something specific that you can talk about. It's almost scripting, but it's healthier. I like what he did. Dynamically, he was directly responding to Justin's comment by turning it around. Jamie's comment directly followed the content of the immediately prior comment.

GD: It would help to have a visual picture of Jamie. He always showed up for group with food smeared all over his face and shirt. He was always covered with catsup, like Pigpen in the *Peanuts* comic strip. For Jamie to make this comment, given his uncommon appearance, was pretty remarkable. He was somehow very appealing despite his personal hygiene.

MN: That would be why he conveyed a sense of hope rather than despair. I like that he brought in playing freeze-tag. He was saying that you could titrate how much you try, or how much you can tolerate, being with others because you can "freeze" it, like freezing the frame of a film. You can put the TV on "Pause," give yourself a break, and then return to the interpersonal world when you are ready. He was using a metaphor that may have seemed as if it were a non-sequitur, but it really wasn't. It was actually quite insightful. His approach also gave instrumentality to the youngster so he could feel less at the mercy of the others.

GD: Taking the issue further, freeze-tag gives children a moment not only to pause in their interactive capacity, but also to be in a space where they can look at others and process the affective cues. They can stop the interaction and back away momentarily to collect themselves in order to continue interacting. It's helpful to the kind of child who can't temperamentally sustain engagement.

Therapist: Is there anybody in here who is a shy person or who knows somebody who was?

Jamie: Of course we were shy when we were babies.

Therapist: So nobody in here is shy and doesn't know how to speak up to friends? Do you know anybody who is?

Oliver: I kind of know what it's like to be called names a lot. It doesn't really have anything to do with what I do at break time. If you have problems like that and they call you names, try doing this. Talk to a teacher about this. That's what I did and we started a group at my school formed of kids who are called names. I used to not say anything and I'm pretty proud of you (the letter-writer) for telling someone about it because that's what I did. Only one in like fifty people have bravery to say that they've been called names and they can do something about it and make it stop. It builds your self-esteem and then it's easier for you to shrug it off. By the way, if one of the kids that's making fun of you is a new kid, like with me at my school, it's mostly because they want to make friends and they just see the first person who has glasses and dismisses them as a dweeb or a nerd. He's probably calling you names so that he can make the other kids think that he's tough and has friends.

GD: Oliver had talked before about the group that he had formed at school. That group was very meaningful to him.

MN: He didn't experience it as making him weird or weirder. He experienced it as helpful.

GD: He felt that it built his self-esteem, which helped him face the name-calling that he was subjected to. He frequently brought up how wearing glasses bothered him: being called "Four eyes." He was a very handsome boy who felt that he was an outlier.

MN: Most kids who wear glasses do not get teased, so the fact that he did suggests that there was something else about him. Also, he was speaking as if the letter-writer were right in the room. He was reaching out and being inclusive. There was nothing that the therapist could have said about it at that moment other than to be aware of it. Oliver clearly had the capacity to reach out and care. He had an appealing empathic quality.

GD: I like how he said, "Only one in fifty people have bravery like that!" It would make me feel wonderful if I were a child like this and heard this advice.

Therapist: What I was thinking about is that Mike started out shy, talking like this and looking down at his shoes, then kids started calling him The Mumbler and dweeb, and next thing you know, he's looking down even more at his shoes.

GD: I thought it would be helpful to paint a picture of what Mike might look like—the body posture, the voice, and the non-verbal cues he was putting out.

MN: There is a vicious cycle that he had gotten himself into. He acted shy; he behaved in a certain maladaptive manner; the situation got worse; then he did it again, and it kept going on and on. This group might have been capable of discerning this, particularly since they stayed on cue throughout the session. Their process hadn't moved them away.

GD: Because of this group's functioning, I thought that I could bring in the causality, the larger perspective of the problem. There was genuineness to the group; they were available and so I thought they could do this.

Justin: Michael has to be able to ignore them.

Therapist: That's hard to do when you have low self-esteem.

Justin: If he ignores them then his self-esteem could go up. He needs to find the occasional friend to make a friendship.

Therapist: That's the point you keep on making and I like that.

Oliver: It's me, again, Oliver (taking the mike). What Georgia said is kind of like the sound of a microphone and holding it up against a speaker. It becomes louder and louder. The only way to stop it from making noise is by turning it off. You're making your self-esteem lower and lower and lower. Now try to make the self-esteem meter go on.

MN: This group used a lot of metaphor. They worked with language in a different way than the other groups, showing that they were able to function at higher level.

GD: In contrast to the girls' groups we just talked about, these boys showed a beautiful soul. They were very touching. Outwardly, one would never have expected this when you saw them coming in, muscling one another, and doing noogies on each other's heads. What they were saying to one another was very poignant and touching.

MN: That was the personality of this group. These boys had been doing this all along. Each group has a personality style, just like we think about how each individual patient has his own personality style. Each group has its own rules for how much they speak about, the permission they give one another to share personal information, the warmth they give one another, and the depth they will go into.

GD: This was a very caring group that reached out to one another.

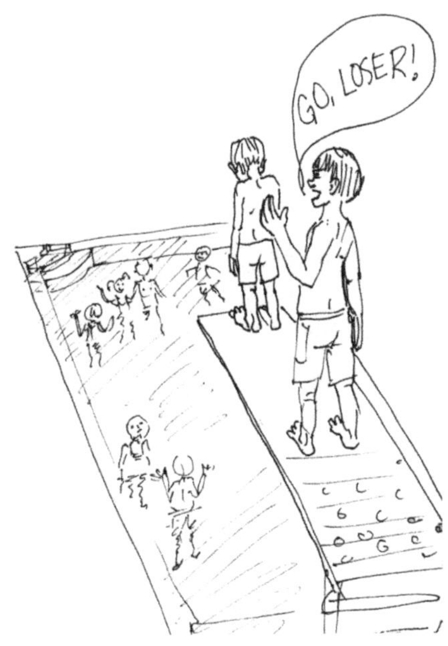

Boys' Group #1

Javier: I don't really have advice, but I usually have the same problems a lot of time. I eat lunch alone and I don't really talk to people. I do have some friends at school; actually I have a lot of friends at school because the class is so small. The thing is, when I eat lunch with a larger group, they either try to engage me in large amounts of conversation or pull pranks on me. One or two pranks are OK, I can live with that. But more than that starts to bug me. The noise level gets me.

MN: This is a great example of a child whose constitutional problems, and how he was overwhelmed by noise, affected his interpersonal functioning. This, in turn, had an impact on his self-esteem. The two became intertwined.

Javier: I have an unfortunately long and complicated life with noise because I live with a younger brother who thinks his greatest purpose in the world is to talk and talk and talk. Then he talks some more. Apparently he even talks and screams in his sleep.

Therapist: Javier, you're bringing up something that maybe Michael has never thought of. Your desire to be alone is not necessarily because you don't have something to say, but because of the noise and the conversation. Is that it?

GD: I chose to follow-through and link the problem of feeling alone and isolated with his constitutional difficulty tolerating noise.

Javier: Sometimes it's just the noise that gets me to back off.

GD: This was nice. He owned his problem and recognized what it did to him.

Therapist: What do you think you could advise so that he could have more company?

Javier: When it gets that noisy, I tend to get claustrophobic.

MN: What he said was that he actually required getting claustrophobic in order to escape the noise. The noise frightened him because it literally hurt his ears. The noise was everywhere. It was coming in on him, as if the noise were walls that were closing in.

GD: I think that's how he perceived it. The group room was small and it could often get very noisy with six boys in it.

Tyrone: When you have recess or break, and everyone is doing something and you're all alone, then join in with what everyone else is doing. Then after a while, then people will acknowledge that you're there. I saw people in my class doing that.

GD: That was a nice observation.

MN: Tyrone was giving advice to the letter-writer and moving away from the noise/claustrophobic problem. He brought in a way to cope with it and became, for the moment, the group's therapist.

GD: Tyrone was very interesting. He was a high-functioning Asperger's youngster who used his visual observation skills to teach himself how people interact with one another.

Henry: It's going to be really hard for you to be accepted in a large group because they already see you as their own personal entertainment. They're already mean to you and they're probably not going to want you playing with them.

GD: This was true. Henry was ostracized at school and was very alone.

MN: He was speaking of hopelessness and describing how humiliating it was to be teased in public for the personal entertainment of others.

GD: I felt very sad when he said that and saw the effect of his comment on the group. The group was fizzling out before my eyes and I needed to regroup them.

Therapist: How many boys in this group consider themselves shy? Javier does. Who considers himself outgoing? Sometimes some of you. There's nothing wrong with being shy. Javier said an interesting thing about himself. He's lucky enough to be in a small class so he gets to know people even though he's shy.

GD: I thought it was important to comment on how the environment can help a child who is shy to make connections with others.

Therapist: Not everyone has that advantage. It makes sense that if it's helped him because he doesn't like a lot of noise, it's good to look for opportunities where you can be in smaller groups that aren't so noisy and a little easier to get to know people.

Javier: I'm in eighth grade at my school, the highest grade and the biggest one too. In the whole eighth grade there are forty-five people. The whole school is 140 kids so it's a small school.

Therapist: You've been fortunate to be in that situation.

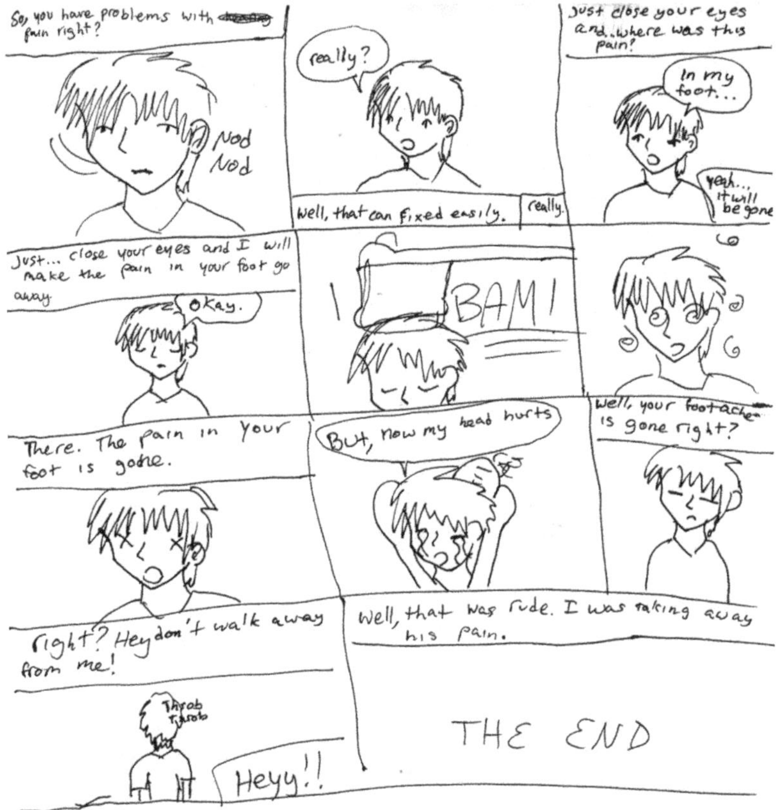
So, you have problems with pain right?
Nod Nod
really?
Well, that can fixed easily.
really.
Just close your eyes and..where was this pain?
In my foot...
yeah... it will be gone
Just... close your eyes and I will make the pain in your foot go away
Okay.
BAM!
There. The pain in your foot is gone.
But, now my head hurts
Well, your footache is gone right?
right? Hey don't walk away from me!
Throb Throb
Heyy!!
Well, that was rude. I was taking away his pain.
THE END

Suggested Activities

1. Ask children to generate scenarios when they have been teased. Role-play situations and generate different strategies that may be used to help the children with being teased.
2. Make masks out of cardboard to depict a character who each child would like to be. Another variation might be to make a hat out of newspapers or construction paper to depict a side of themselves. For groups with fine motor difficulties, provide an assortment of interesting hats. Ask children to select one that depicts something about their personality, then create a story.

References

Brooks, B., & Siegel, P. M. (1996). *The scared child: Helping kids overcome traumatic events.* New York: Wiley.

Carey, W. B., & McDevitt, S. C. (1995). *Coping with children's difficult temperament.* New York: Basic Books.

DeGangi, G. A., & Kendall, A. (2008). *Effective parenting for the hard-to-manage child.* New York: Routledge.

Greenspan, S. I., & Salmon, J. (1996). *The challenging child: Understanding, raising, and enjoying the five 'difficult' types of children.* Cambridge, MA: Perseus Publishing.

Klass, P., & Costello, E. (2003). *Quirky kids: Understanding and helping your child who doesn't fit in—when to worry and when not to worry.* New York: Ballantine Books.

CHAPTER 14
Tell Me Master What to Do! I'll Do Anything ... To Be Popular Like You

Children often yearn to become a member of the most popular group at school and sometimes will do anything to make that happen. They might be willing to compromise personal values to be included. One youngster, for example, might command and exploit another child to steal, lie, or give them the answers on a test. Some boys might be ordered to hand over their best toys with the promise that these acts will gain them popularity. In the end, the child loses out, is placed in a subservient role, and often ends up being ridiculed. Unfortunately, such social failures do not prevent vulnerable children from trying these same approaches over and over. Learning healthy ways to assert oneself with peers, while remaining true to oneself, is at the heart of the matter, a task for all people, children, and adults (Heaney & Israel, 2002; Pipher, 1994). The following letter was written to help the groups explore the price that some friendships have for children, while also evoking the related issues of identity and social alienation.

> *Dear Kids' Club,*
>
> I used to be a real outcast socially and had zero friends, but this year I figured out a good solution to the problem. There are some really cool, popular kids who I really admire. I have wanted to be part of their group for so long. They are good at sports, wear cool clothes, and everyone wishes they could be like them. The two kids who are the coolest, Robin and Jamie, have started to ask me to do things for them, then tell me that I am the greatest. I love that! Finally, someone is liking me. The only bad part is that I sometimes do things for them that I'm not sure are such a good idea. They took off from the playground during recess and ran around to the parking lot to do something. When the teacher came by, I was supposed to say that they were inside in the bathroom. One time they asked me to go in some kids' backpacks in the locker room and take any money I could find. They want me to sneak into Mr. Thompson's room, the science teacher, and see if I can steal a copy of the test that we're getting on Friday. I haven't done it yet but if I don't do it, they said they would stop liking me.

This is my only chance for friends and I don't want to lose being with Robin and Jamie. They said I have to keep doing what they ask as an initiation into their club. I'm really confused and not sure what to do. I don't want to blow it. What do you think?

Signed,
Walter, a Wannabee Cool Kid
(Chelsea in girls' version)

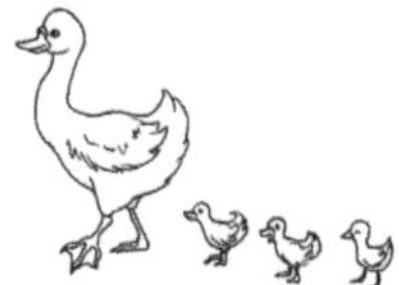

MN: This letter addresses multiple issues—social isolation, alienation, and self-identity.

GD: Even though this letter appears in this section of letters having to do with interpersonal effectiveness, it also relates to how the ability to affiliate appropriately with peers often hinges on the security of a child's identity and his capacity to overcome barriers to feeling isolated.

MN: "What is the price of belonging, and who am I?"

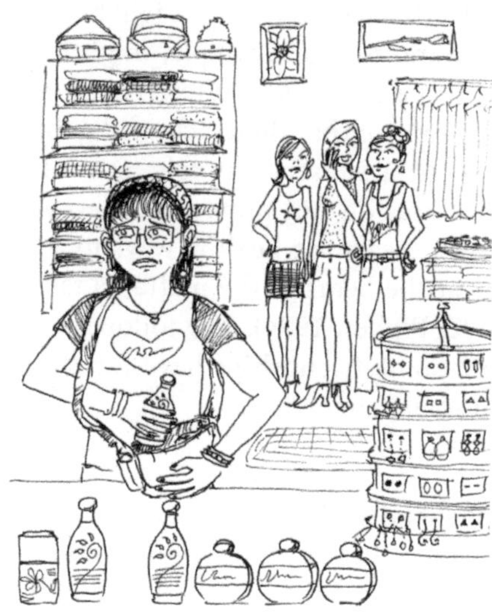

Girls' Group #3

Gillian: If you're sad and mad that you have to steal so many things, don't worry. You should just talk to your teachers and the principal about what's going on and they can probably help you with whatever you need.

MN: Gillian identified some of the more global feelings involved. It was a nice start, although a bit simplistic.

GD: I don't think she had really connected to the letter's content yet.

Deborah: I know what these people are doing and I've read about it. It's called "hazing." It's what people do where they make you do a lot of bad things to you to get in their club. I know how hard it is not to have any friends. If people are doing this, they aren't really friends. They're taking advantage of you. It's not like they're giving anything up. You shouldn't be friends with them.

Therapist: These aren't real friends at all.

MN: Deborah took care of the group process problem. She moved beyond Gillian's simplistic response and got closer to the letter's core. What you did was mirror Deborah's very clear expression of exploitation. She shared, from the heart, that she had difficulty making connections with others.

GD: I loved that she was able to reveal to the group that not having friends was hard for her. She was just beginning to bring this up in the group sessions. At the time that this group occurred, we were doing a project. All the girls had to build something collaboratively inside of a single box. It could have been anything they wanted to make the inside of the box become. Deborah couldn't get past the fact that the group didn't like her idea.

MN: She would have experienced her social isolation right then. Her "real world" difficulty was being enacted in the group. She then had an in vivo laboratory in which to work on the issue. This is one of the benefits of group therapy; you have the members' social problems right in the room.

GD: Deborah wanted to build a town from the past with a synagogue in it. None of the girls were buying her idea. They wanted to make a horse stable with stalls and a riding pasture which was very much like girls this age. Deborah just could not join the others' theme. She was so stuck on making her synagogue that I remember encouraging her to go ahead and make that and then see if there was a way to bridge the horse story with the synagogue story.

MN: "The Synagogue Riding School." I'm treating this too lightly. Deborah, through her rigidity, was participating in her own exclusion. She was, on the other hand, trying to assert part of her identity.

GD: All I could think about right then was how rigid Deborah was in her thinking and how this affected her relatedness. Even on a gestural level, she was unable to make the needed connection to her peers. So, I was glad that she brought up, in response to this letter, that she didn't have any friends.

MN: There was an issue in this group moment about identity and defensive function. In the description you just gave about the project, the other kids were working with their age-appropriate interests. Deborah, though, felt compelled to bring in something from her background that was more internal and not really shareable in the context of this project.

GD: Deborah couldn't understand the difference between one internal aspect of herself, her Jewishness, and anything else about herself that could have been shared and accepted. Some of the other girls were indeed Jewish but this really wasn't a subject much on their minds.

MN: Deborah held on to only one part of herself; it served as a defense against her anxiety about being known by others, and being with others. I also wonder if the horses troubled her; horses for girls are often a symbol of power, particularly of male power. The implication of aggression would have been scary for her.

GD: During this project, even Gillian, the girl with cerebral palsy, was able to join the horse theme. But not Deborah. And the other girls simply weren't interested in Jewishness. Deborah could not manage this and so she isolated herself, resentfully.

MN: I think that they wanted to join on the level of other interests, which made sense at this age and demonstrated a greater capacity, or potential, for developing and maintaining relationships.

Ashley: Maybe they really feel like you and they'd rather be popular. They are just using you. You can probably find other people who are a real friend.

Kendra: I don't have this problem, but it's better to choose friends who are real friends.

MN: I wonder why Ashley had to disavow this problem, since the issue was not whether one had this problem or not. Perhaps she was anxious about what it would be like to feel alienated and not have friends. The letter might actually have frightened her more than she was saying.

GD: Kendra was adopted and bi-racial. Her parents were Caucasian. There were three adopted children in the family. One was blond, blue-eyed and very pretty. The other child was also African-American. Kendra's identity problems ran deep. She was not really included in her family and she felt like an outlier, as if she didn't belong to her family. She also had gender identity issues that showed up in her appearance. Every week she'd show up at group with a baseball cap on and sports apparel. I would often look at her and think, "If I didn't know this child, I would think that she was a boy." It's interesting that she disavowed this problem but focused on how she did not have this other specific difficulty of being coerced to do things. I agree with you. She was distancing herself, telling the group: "Don't go there!"

Therapist: That's right. It's better to have fewer friends who are genuine and nice than a lot of friends who are mean.

Ashley: You don't want to be friends with those girls just because they're including you. They're doing it for the wrong reasons.

Kendra: Last word of advice—don't be their friends.

MN: Was Kendra being charming or was she actually trying to convey, in "group process-speak"—"That's enough!"

GD: It was a "that's enough" response.

Boys' Group #3

Oliver: In the letters that we've gotten in this boys' group, a lot of people suffer from the same problems that I do. I have to agree with you (the letter-writer). When you're the outcast and have zero friends, you kind of do anything that you would do to be popular. But when they tell you to steal stuff, even if you want to be popular, you can't do it. The advice that I give to you is: don't do it! Do the same thing that I'm doing. Try to start a school group for the kids that feel that they're the outcasts. There may not be a chance and it may not happen. Maybe you and your fellow outcasts maybe won't become outcasts anymore because you'll become friends. That's what I'm doing at my school. I already set up a log, a teacher, and a room. You can just do it if you follow in my footsteps. At first it's really hard. You're just writing the letter and that's really a good head start. Keep on going, man. I feel his pain.

GD: What Oliver said was so appealing. I loved his response.

MN: He was on-target and it was really a very good idea to put together a group of other outcasts. If outcasts can come together, they become "Former Outcasts." They become "in" because they are together. It could be a group of Capital M "Misfits" who no longer are misfits because they have peers who are like them and who do like each other. They have an affiliation.

GD: Yes. They would have each other. Eventually, Oliver became perceived as belonging to a group, rather than the loner who sat by himself with no one to talk to.

MN: He was also being very resourceful. He had served this resourceful function for the group before.

GD: Yes, he had, but he had also served the function of bringing forward very dark thoughts about committing suicide. He was the only boy who went to that dark place. The group tolerated it well, allowing him the space to express those troubling, even frightening feelings. Basically, he had been given permission by the group to have those thoughts and still be part of the group. The group didn't distance itself from him or ostracize him.

MN: Although I don't like to stereotype, boys generally do have more difficulty expressing feelings. These boys, however, were able to function in a way that was emotional and tolerant of the other group members' feelings, despite feeling uncomfortable. A therapist must ask: "What was it about this group's constitution that helped create this good chemistry? What was it about this group that permitted it to tolerate affect so consistently?"

GD: When we look at the constellation of this group we have Leo and Justin who had Asperger's syndrome, and Jamie who had social learning disabilities. Oliver was the only one without Asperger's, but rather severe anxiety with depression. He was a great catalyst in this group. He worked better in this group than he might have in a group of other anxious boys.

Leo: This is Leo. My advice is don't steal the test, even if you really want to know the answers; because you don't know a lot of the stuff on it, you'll study. My advice is to find new friends and get out of the club. I think you should find someone who has the same interests as you. One day you'll have friends. This Robin and Jamie sound like real bullies. My advice is stay away from them. If you find a new friend, you may get new friends. If you hang around with Robin and Jamie on the other hand, you'll probably never make any more friends.

MN: Leo's comment seemed disconnected from the general discussion. It illustrates the Theory-of-Mind that Asperger's children struggle to develop: they have trouble understanding and interpreting the motivation and intentions of other people. Instead, they are concrete and miss the intended communication of others. Often, they simply don't get it and have to be taught.

Justin: That Robin and Jamie are really false friends, not true friends. You are a total servant of them. You shouldn't do the things they want you to do because you'll probably end up with a bad school record if you get caught doing all these things. Of course they'll dump you in the end. Do this for your own sake. Oliver is right in finding other outcasts. Or try to find a new friend that you can befriend. Do your best.

Jamie: Here's some good advice. Drop some money in your own backpack and show it to them. Then bring the teacher over and bust them. Tell them they're stealing. Find some other friends by playing sports.

GD: He was basically saying, "Frame them!"

MN: The idea of framing them is in its way cute from a child this age, but Jamie's really not talking about the relationship that the letter-writer has with these boys who are exploiting him. He's talking about revenge.

GD: I think he was sincerely thinking that this was somehow a good idea.

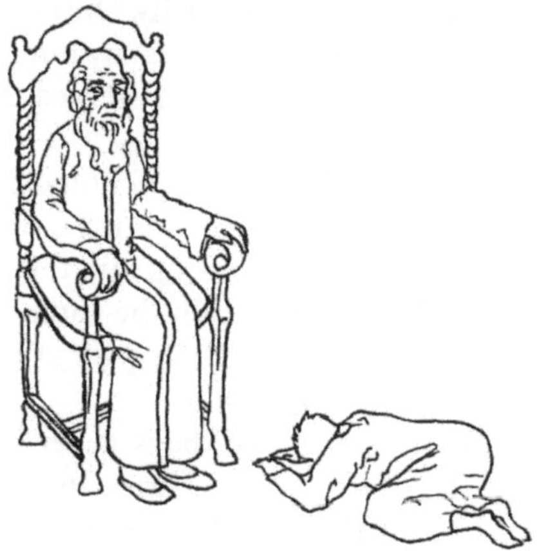

Boys' Group #1

Henry: They're not your friends! They are never going to be your friends! They're just using you! They're making you do things so that they don't get in trouble and you do. End of story.

Jacob: As you said, they're just being your false friends so that they can get your stuff. If you keep on doing that, they'll probably keep making you do more stuff. Eventually you'll get caught and get blamed.

GD: I was very proud of Jacob for speaking about the falseness of these people because it was very difficult to get him to be genuine about his own feelings. He usually acted like the comedian Jerry Lewis. Something in this letter pushed him to be more real than he usually was. Manuel, who spoke next, had just joined the group.

Manuel: My name is Manuel, AKA Manny the Mouse. Those guys are complete jerks so ignore them because if you get in trouble, your chance of being popular goes down the drain as well. Forget what they say. They are wrong. If they get a copy of the test and it's a State test, they can go to jail. Also, you can get in trouble for aiding and abetting a felon.

MN: This was not really an off-topic response; it was purely practical and didn't attend to feelings. The writer wrote the letter because of his feelings. Manuel was new to the group, so we don't know if this is how he truly viewed the world, a social misunderstanding, or if he was experiencing anxiety about trying to find his way into the group. If this comment represented his world-view, he sounds like a frightened child given to catastrophizing.

GD: Interestingly, I'd been working with Manuel for several years before he first entered this group. He was in ninth grade then and had gotten himself into some terrible trouble at school because of social misunderstandings. He'd been accused of stalking a girl, staring at her while they were in drama club. He had taken manicure sets to school in his wallet and the principal suspended him for it. He explained it innocently: "I was just showing another kid this manicure set in my wallet." When I replied, "You know that sharp objects are not allowed at your school. What were you doing showing someone this?" He responded, "It was in my wallet and I just showed him." He missed some serious connections of logic and consequences. He was a very bright child.

MN: His idiosyncratic reasoning was notable in this comment. He put the manicure set in his wallet and he couldn't articulate why he did it. (I also don't understand what a ninth grade boy would be doing with a manicure set in the first place.) He was acting without thinking and then of course he couldn't explain it after the fact.

Javier: The trick is you'll be the felon as far as anybody else is concerned because how do they know that someone else got you to do it.

Manuel: You'll harass them out.

GD: Here was another example of Manuel's off-center thinking. He was continuing despite Javier's more sensible, though dramatic, comment. I thought that Manuel was trying to stay with the flow of the group, but just couldn't do it because his thinking was so odd.

Henry: Javier stole the microphone from me. One thing you can do is tell them what they're doing to you.

GD: It was striking that he mentioned that Javier had stolen the microphone from him, especially since the theme is being taken advantage of, being exploited.

MN: At that moment, the group was partly acting-out the problems described in the letter. In its way, Henry' comment was part of the flow of the group.

Therapist: What do you think this guy can do instead to make friends?

Henry: First option is tell the teacher but tell them not to tell those kids that you told on them. Otherwise they'll kill you. Second option: make a fake test, that's kind of hard. Another option would be find some other friends. Those people are not your friends. It's not easy. You have to find somebody with a common interest as you. You really need to find friends.

MN: Henry got the concept that these boys are not true friends. In this part of the conversation there was a lot of underlying aggression. They were talking about payback and going to jail. Outside the group, Manuel acted out later, to be sure that the group would know that there was indeed a degree of aggression present in the issues described in the letter. Sharp objects from the school's point-of-view are weapons and he knew it. This letter evoked underlying aggressive fantasy in some of these boys. I wonder if there was also a degree of identification with the exploitation of friends even though they were talking about giving advice to the sufferer.

GD: Except for Jacob, these boys would have had difficulty acting out aggression in overt ways. They would have found more passive ways to be aggressive.

MN: Their passivity may have been an inhibition of aggression. Some temperamental or constitutional factors are likely to have affected the way in which they expressed aggression, but I don't think it accounted for all of it.

Tyrone: If you try to steal the test and the teacher saw you, the teacher might fail you. You could get a zero on the test because you were trying to cheat. The other people who told you to do it wouldn't fail, but you would.

MN: There might have been a temptation here for the therapist to say something, but this group was functioning well and running on its own by this time in the session. From a group dynamic framework, the therapist didn't need to say anything. One of the goals of group therapy is to have the group learn to do the group work on its own as much as possible.

Henry: Here's a fourth option. Tell them that you looked in all the drawers of the teacher's desk and you couldn't find the test, then make them go in there and get them caught by a teacher.

Javier: These people are not your friends; they're using you. You're not going to make friends by doing stupid things or wrong things. That's not friendship. It's slavery. It's servitude. There's a difference between someone who compliments you and is your master and someone who compliments you and is your real friend. A real friend won't ask you to do something that is wrong. You mentioned those boys running off to the parking lot. My question to you is: "What were they doing there?" You probably don't want to find out what they were doing.

MN: That was a helpful, focused comment; it also kept the group going by ignoring what Henry said about setting a trap for the exploiters. Javier knew that Henry's comment was unhelpful and so he proceeded with something that made more sense.

GD: Despite Javier's Asperger's, he had learned through strong moral fiber and excellent cognitive reasoning how social relationships work. We can hear the script that must have run in his head all the time about how relationships should work. I was very proud of him.

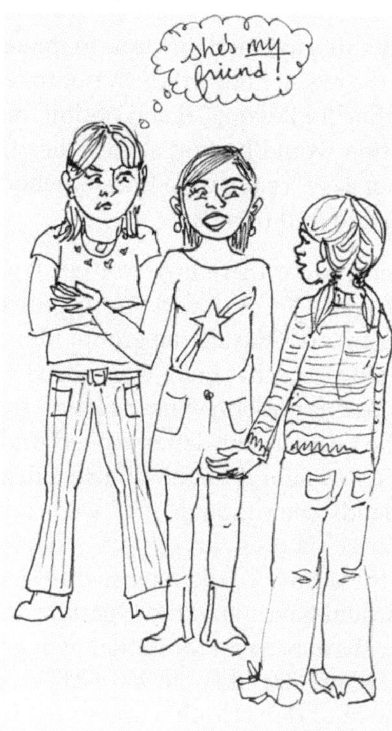

Girls' Group #5

Nadia: If your friends tell you to steal something and try to sneak it, don't listen to them because you don't want to get in trouble.

GD: Nadia was a lot like the child in this letter: primed for exploitation by others in order to become accepted. She had been taunted at school to do things such as climb under the bathroom stalls, lock them, and then climb out.

Nadia: Once I tried that and I got caught. Say that you don't really want to do that, but you still want to be their friend. Don't do anything about stealing, but do other stuff.

GD: Nadia did not quite understand that she was being made into a servant or that she was being coerced into doing things that she shouldn't be doing. She understood the rule—"Thou shalt not steal. Stealing is wrong."

MN: This is a concrete thought, strictly about behavior, but she didn't understand the social interaction or the social meaning of what was occurring between the exploiters and the exploited. She was also not attending to the feelings of desperation that a child might have, enough so that she would be willing to do almost anything in order to be accepted.

Therapist: It sounds like you were in this position before and that you know exactly what Chelsea is up against. Did you do it to win friendships?

GD: I decided to make a comment to lure Nadia into the discussion rather than saying something that she might construe to be judgmental. I also wanted to see if she could understand the social desperation of the letter-writer, but I wanted to do it gently.

MN: This is an example of when it would not be helpful for the therapist to offer a highly clarifying statement to the group as a whole. Nadia's was the first response to the letter. It started the group. So at such a time, the therapist should aim on focusing the discussion. It's exactly the time the therapist should speak in a facilitating way.

GD: Since Nadia had done things like the letter-writer had done, I wanted to support her in bringing it up in the group and to let her know that we would be nonjudgmental. I wanted the group to know that we supported them in sharing thoughts and feelings and that they would not to be judged by me or by the other girls.

Nadia: No. This friend, Warren, he told me to go into Miss Collins' desk and take things. He said, "Just do it fast and get out of here." So we did, and Warren got out before I did. I got caught and it wasn't fair.

GD: I didn't know about that incident. There were so many instances when Nadia showed poor social judgment. Nadia was adopted from Russia, and this was an important issue, because it related to her own sense of acceptability. She had wonderful parents but developing a solid attachment with anyone had been difficult, as it often may be with adopted children. She would become desperate to be liked and do things hoping for an attachment, or hoping for what she perceived as a secure relationship.

Brittany: Well, you really shouldn't hang out with them if they're making you do this. You should hang out with regular friends instead of popular friends even though you may want to be in with the cool crowd. You can make up friends yourself and pretend that they're popular. I do this sometimes when I'm all alone at recess. I pretend I'm in a really cool outfit.

MN: That's close to bizarre. She began much more grounded with the material than she concluded. Her anxiety got the better of her thought-processing. Was she describing getting lost in her own head and dissociating as a way of dealing with the pain of exclusion?

GD: I think she was. She pretended quite a bit that something was happening when it really was not. I don't know if it was dissociation, or a more straightforward strong defense against feeling excluded.

MN: Brittany's response raises an important group process question for the therapist. As the group continued, how might we understand her function within it, and how might the therapist both help her and at the same time use her off-kilter material to help the group? It was possible that she was the spokesperson, unfortunately, for a group tendency to dissociate when things got rough. Or the group could come to observe what she was doing and learn that it would be maladaptive rather than useful. It's particularly important that the therapist be able to balance content with process.

GD: Brittany's adoptive mother would frequently dissociate when distressed. This placed Brittany in the role of taking care of her mother, something she really didn't have the equipment to do, or even to tolerate. Her mother was also teaching her, by the way she behaved, that dissociation was appropriate.

MN: Brittany had the additional problem of needing to identify with a very damaged primary maternal object, creating a damaged introject.

Melissa: I've been in this position a few times and I have to say, it's better to have good friends than to get in trouble. I have friends now who are not popular, but they're nicer than the popular kids. The popular kids are the meanest and they get the worst grades. Being a good friend with kids who are nice and have things in common with you is the most important thing.

Therapist: How did you get from being with the kids who were making you do things to having good friends?

Melissa: I just made up excuses to them. "I just want to go play with these kids, and I might play with you tomorrow." "I just want to have some alone time right now."

Therapist: It's good to know how you figured out how to get off the hook with them.

MN: It's a good solution: keep making excuses and eventually they'll lose interest and stop bugging you. This was an example of the therapist and one group member continuing the ongoing process of the group, rather than disrupting it.

Brooke: What you can do is say to them, "Even though you're popular, you don't have good grades and you don't have a good attitude." Even though they're the most popular kids in the school, and they look cool and act cool, they're so superficial. Maybe they're a clique. I think you should not go to them because they're superficial. They say stuff like, "Oh my God, I broke a nail. I have to go get a manicure now." Make some other friends. Good luck.

Therapist: What you're all saying is that you want a real friend who you can trust and who will really listen to you.

GD: Brooke's spin on this was interesting. She moved from being one of the most superficial, narcissistic children I had ever seen, to one who became capable of attachment. However, in the group it was only to me, not the other children. None of the girls liked her.

MN: Did she eventually develop the capacity for empathy?

GD: It took probably three years of group therapy before I saw signs of empathy developing in her. It eventually became genuine, but at first it seemed rehearsed, "the proper thing to do."

Girls' Group #1

Rosa: Maybe you should just ignore them. The bullies are trying to get you out of school. Ignore their ideas. Find some real friends that can talk to you and do things with you.

MN: Rosa did an interesting thing here. She labeled what was actually happening in the letter. It wasn't a long explanation, but she did label it as bullying. She was the first person in all these groups who had actually used the word. She started the whole discussion quite eloquently—"These are not your friends. They're bullying you. And you're being exploited." It's by using the word "bullying" that she accomplished it. This is an example of when the therapist must really "micro-listen," pick this up and make good use of it during the ensuing session.

GD: I liked that she brought up that it would be important to ignore the bullies' ideas. Her comments here were really useful.

Crystal: I think that you should just ignore them and tell the teacher what they've been doing.

GD: The process continued. Crystal followed-up what Rosa had said.

Mallory: I don't want to be mean. I don't know.

GD: Mallory was saying that she didn't know how to set a limit and be forceful with others when asked to do something she didn't want to do. She also continued the group along its' process.

MN: Mallory's comment was heartfelt and personally exposing. Some groups of children this age have troubling tolerating such self-exposure.

GD: They do, but it's really because they sometimes don't quite understand it. It goes right over their heads. That's what happened in this group.

Therapist: What were you thinking of saying to her?

Mallory: I think that Chelsea is sort of crazy to think that those people could be her friends.

Therapist: She doesn't understand what is happening. Chelsea wants friends so desperately that she is willing to do anything. How can she get out of that problem so that she doesn't do something wrong just to get a friend?

Mallory: I think she shouldn't be friends with them.

Therapist: But she wants friends. She said to me, "These friends are better than no friends." So I told her, "let's find out what other girls think about your situation." How can she find friends who aren't mean? Have any of you found a way to find a friend who isn't mean? (No response.)

GD: I used the word "mean" because Mallory used it. I thought using the technique of reflection was very important at this moment in the group.

MN: The lack of response from the group, the change in the trajectory of the group process, came from the heartfelt comment, "I don't want to be mean." Mallory got emotionally stuck. I don't know if she had become the spokesperson for the group and that they were all stuck, or if her exposed honesty was shutting them down. That would be a shame because she could be an asset to this group's development over time.

GD: I can picture Mallory when she made that statement, with her head down, her hair falling over her face, with wringing hands. At the same time, Mallory was the girl who brought a large rope noose to group to share. She would bring the rope and ask the girls if they would like to see her tie a noose. She talked with me in her individual treatment about her desire to kill her stepmother and how she would do it with knives. This came out in an individual session shortly after this group. I think the group discussion assisted her in being able to talk about it. I asked: "Is your stepmother in danger from you?" and she said, "Maybe. I've thought about killing her when she's asleep in her bed." I replied, "Then I need to warn her that you have these thoughts. We need to be sure all the knives in the house are far away from you because you're having a thought that's dangerous." I remember saying, "Do you want to be mean to your stepmother?" and she said, "No, I'm not mean. But she is mean and hateful to me because she married my father. That's who is mean." She had a misattribution about causality related to who was the mean person and she couldn't own these disturbing, aggressive thoughts. When she would bring out the noose, she acted in an almost depersonalized way, as if it were not she who was holding it.

MN: I believe that she was relying on projection in an attempt to figure out just who was "mean." She's told us that "I don't want to be mean," but that is only half the story. She failed to understand her own ambivalence about aggression: she could accept it in others but needed to rationalize it, depersonalize it, or simply ignore it in herself. This leads me to the same question—"What was the function that Natalie served in the group?"

GD: One of the limits of group psychotherapy is that sometimes it is necessary to have information available only from other ongoing modalities of treatment. Sometimes these other modalities aren't in place for some youngsters who need it. If I hadn't known this child through individual psychotherapy and family work, I wouldn't have had the whole story available to me so that I could interpret her statement about meanness in a more holistic way. For this reason, sometimes it's good to know the child in multiple settings.

MN: The unfortunate difficulty is that it is too often infeasible for a youngster to be in more than one treatment modality. The other problem is that the therapist must be a good prognosticator and have a good sense of who requires multi-modal treatment and who doesn't.

Abby: Try to ignore the tricks.

GD: She went back to Rosa's first comment—wrapping the group session up. This is a good example of the group's need to come full circle before stopping.

Suggested Activities

1. Provide a piece of paper to each child in the group. Ask them to write down one attribute of another child in the group without saying who they are describing. For example, the child might write down, "Funny, sensitive, caring, bossy, adventurous …." The children then guess whom the child has written about. They can discuss how authentic the description might be, allowing the children to react to who is being described. If this activity is done in a supportive and therapeutic way, it can be very useful in providing feedback to one another while helping the child see how others see them. This requires therapeutic delicacy.
2. Give each child a collection of magnetic sticks and balls to play with. Place some of the magnetic sticks and balls in the center of the table and see if the children make their own construction or add onto the "group" construction. Have each child describe what she built. If they added to the one in the middle, each child can take a turn modifying it and describing what they think it is. This is a good projective activity and one that lends itself to discussing the process of working alone or in a group.

References

Heaney, C. A., & Israel, A. (2002). Social networks and social support. In K. Glanz, F. Lewis, & B. Rimer (Eds.), *Health behavior and health education: Theory, research and practice* (3rd ed., pp. 185–209). San Francisco: Jossey-Bass.

Pipher, M. (1994). *Reviving ophelia: Saving the selves of adolescent girls*. New York: Ballantine Books.

CHAPTER **15**

The Sibling Battleground

Friend or Foe?

Many, if not most, children the ages of those in these groups, find themselves in the midst of a conflict with their brother or sister and have no idea how to extricate themselves. They do not have the tools necessary to negotiate sibling conflict. Often this is the result of residue of earlier sibling rivalry such that current conflicts are informed by old resentments. Sometimes the child provokes his sibling purposely. At other times he unwittingly does things that set the sibling off on a course of irritation and retaliation. There are yet other occasions when the instigations, accusations, and retaliations of sibling rivalry are simply on pernicious automatic pilot. There are children who get ensnared in a conflict which they didn't do anything to instigate. They become inflamed by the situation when their parents blame them for engineering the whole thing, when the sibling was actually the mastermind. Sometimes, sibling wars are more insidious and develop gradually as a result of parental favoritism for the more able or more likable child. In Western culture, sibling rivalry is uncommonly common. The following letter gives voice to one kind of sibling battle.

Dear Kids' Club,

I'm going to get right to my problem. My little sister is the biggest brat! She is always coming into my bedroom and sneaking off with stuff of mine and then she lies about doing it. If I race after her and give her a good wallop, I'm the one who gets in big trouble. When I have friends over, she gets in our face, wants to do what we're doing, and is annoying to the max. She sings stupid songs, grabs our stuff, and follows us around. My parents say, "Give her a break! You're older and it's *your* job to be nice to Mimi."

I try to get back at her if I am forced to let her play games with us, like I'll make sure that she ends up losing the game. Or my friends and I gang up on her to make her life miserable. I can't stand to even look at her face. To top it all off, she is my parents' number one favorite. She gets the best bedroom in the whole house and, the dweeb doesn't even sleep in there. She is such a scaredy-cat that she sleeps in a sleeping bag down by my parents' bedroom.

I say that *I* should get her bedroom and she should have my little rats' nest room. I'm the one with all the project ideas and stuff that needs to spread out. She doesn't even play in her bedroom. My parents say it's all decorated cute for a little girl and we can't switch. Aside from that, I'm sick of the way she gets everything her way and I'm the one who is always getting yelled out. I'd like to send Mimi on a rocket ship to outer space. What should I do to get rid of her?

Signed,
Kevin, the Kid who gets the Shaft
(Kathy in girl's version)

Girl's Group #2

Chelsea: If she's following you around and every once in a while, just stop and she'll bump into you. Or lock your door. And if that doesn't work, put a big spider around your door, or on the door knob and when she opens it, she's going to see the spider dangling over her.

Therapist: But what can Kathy (the letter-writer) do not to get in trouble with her parents?

Chelsea: Tell your parents that she's been following you around and comes into your room and she's the biggest pest that anybody could have for a sister.

MN: Given that Chelsea had an older sister with severe developmental delays, around whom the family revolved, I'm surprised that she did not attend to the obvious favoritism of the parents in the letter. The biggest emotional pull of this letter was the exclusion that the letter-writer felt, even down to living in a rat's nest. He was almost experiencing himself as unwanted. Instead, Chelsea was drawn to seeking revenge.

GD: It's also important to remember that Chelsea's older sister was non-verbal, in a wheelchair, and completely unavailable to Chelsea as a social peer. All the focus in the family was on the sister. The sister was "there but not there," i.e., incomplete. Chelsea was also "there but not there" in the sense that her parents did not experience her as a person, at least as she saw it.

MN: In other words, Chelsea felt unwanted, unfavored, and unseen.

Therapist: She should tell her parents how she feels.

Chelsea: Then you tell your parents that you've been nice to her long enough and that she has not been appreciating you at all.

Briana: You could bug her for something or scare her or do something bad and blame her for it. Or you could get back at her. Make her go play someplace and you do something really bad and tell your parents that she did it. Then she'll get in big trouble and then she'll stop playing with you.

Therapist: Do you think that will work, to set her up to be the one who gets in trouble?

Danielle: Try making a sign for your door that says, "Keep out or I'll tell mom or dad that you're coming in." Lock the door; then when it's OK for them to come into the room, unlock the door. You can get this plastic lock like they have in hotels, and only you, your mom and dad, not your sister, get a copy. A big "NO!" I wanted one of those locks because my brother bugs me when I'm doing my homework.

MN: The essence of this letter is the relationship of the less-favored, more-blamed, child with the parents. As with so much of sibling rivalry, the fear of being the less-preferred child is perceived as being the less-loved child. This is a frightening concept and the girls in the group stayed instead with the more concrete, less troubling issue of revenge, and perhaps some resentment.

GD: The direction of this conversation was interesting. Briana's idea was to sabotage and stab the sister in the back, while Danielle was actually coming up with something that could work, with a limit built into the strategy.

MN: There were two sides to what Briana was saying. She was focusing on things that weren't going to work, like trying to get the parents to blame the sibling whereas the letter-writer's parents have already told her that whenever her sister did things, they would respond by saying things like "Give it over. Get over it. Too bad." Briana was overlooking that and thus she restored the parents' capacity for empathy. Danielle went back to something that might work and did include the parents, to some extent. Her idea was to keep the conflict between the two siblings. The letter had the youngster all alone and without any help. She had to solve this problem all by herself. The parents were not perceived as an asset. They had already told her that it was not a problem and that it was her responsibility to get over it. If she was having a problem with it—"tough."

GD: She was then all alone without a solution and without resources to turn to. The letter-writer was holding a huge volume of anger that couldn't be safely vented in her house because she was the unfavored child.

MN: The girls focused on the issue of resentful anger; they were coming up with aggressive ways to handle the problem, like putting spiders on doorknobs. They were aware of the anger that was purposely not clearly stated in the letter. They were not, however, discussing the sadness of being alone with a problem like this.

Ellen: You could ask your little sister if you could trade places for a day. You could be your sister and she's you. Then you can tell your mom what you're doing and say, "She always acts like this and now you can see what it's really like for me."

GD: Ellen wanted empathy very badly. She wanted her mother to understand what her experience of living with the younger sister was like.

Briana: If you want to get back at her, too, you could tell her that you're going to clean up her room, then make a mess of it. Then tell your parents that she made a big mess in her room.

MN: This was plain sadism—mean-spirited retaliation. However, it did demonstrate how cruelty develops from a severe sibling rivalry situation in which the parents, wittingly or unwittingly, participate.

Annie: You should rearrange the furniture in your own room so it looks bigger and decorate it so that you like your bedroom better.

GD: That was a nice idea to improve the environment if one couldn't change the relational dynamic.

MN: But again, it related to how the letter-writer was in this alone.

GD: It's interesting that Annie said this because it was her style to hold things close to the vest. It was very difficult for her to share anything with anyone. She wrote poetry, but it was only for herself. She understood what it was like to feel alone but, characteristically, she wasn't talking about it.

Latisha: If your parents don't agree with you on the paint color, then you should remind them that it's your room. That's what happened to me and I told them it's not their room and they're not the ones looking at it.

GD: Latisha was responding directly to Annie's comment. This suggests to me that the group members had really been listening to each other and not just offering their comments, one-by-one, to the letter-writer. There was actually more group process occurring than it might seem at first.

MN: And again, the therapist has the difficult task of discerning this kind of subtlety and using her understanding to facilitate the group.

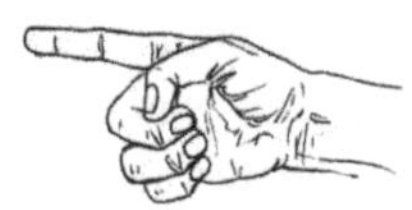

Boys' Group #1

Henry: I know what that's like.

MN: I'll bet he did! I like Henry's ready ability to empathize with the letter-writer. It was a nice beginning to the group.

Therapist: Do you have any solutions?
Henry: No solutions.
Therapist: There's no solution to the bratty little sister?
Henry: Not if you talk to her personally and she doesn't listen to you.
Therapist: So what do you do about your bratty little sister? This will really help Kevin.

MN: Here was a nice example of the therapist having decided to trust the group, believing that with only minimal prompting, a useful process would follow.

GD: I personalized my response to Henry in order to bring him into the room with the problem he had with his own sister. I felt a strong sense of how sad, alone, and depleted Henry felt, and I believed that the group could help him.

Henry: You have to talk to her about the problem and do something nice to her.
Therapist: Kind of like if you're nice to her, then she's nice to you.
Henry: Now she's eight years old and she's still annoying but it's better than before.

MN: Henry had not yet revealed that he had a "real self" behind what he was saying. He offered a hopeless sigh. That airless sigh suggested to me that the affect he was experiencing was too much and that he needed to dissociate it, separate the feeling from the words.

GD: I had a feeling that was similar to letting the air out of a balloon. It felt emotionally limited. I thought Henry felt demoralized and incapable of being an active agent in his life. He just felt stuck with this bratty sister and that he wouldn't be listened to by anyone. My counter-transference was to his loneliness. I really felt for him.

Jacob: There is one solution I know of but it's probably not the best one, but bug your room and put a video camera there so you can tell if your sister came in. Replay the video and if you want to make it look worse, then do a little editing.

GD: That was so like Jacob! Clever, impish, with a touch of the devil.

MN: As therapist in-the-moment, I would have wondered if his humorous riff could have helped the group process or not. Sometimes comments like Jacob's are a manifestation of defensive avoidance, but sometimes they are truly facilitative. Often in a group, timing is everything. The same comment might serve a different function if offered at a different time. In fact, here it was facilitative . . . but only after a while.

Therapist: Remember what he said was that he does a lot of stuff and he's sick and tired of this. How do I take care of this problem and not get in trouble?

Jacob: Show the parents the movie about this. It may cost a lot of money and you'd have to keep it on all the time. You can also do something in your sister's room when she's not in there and get her back.

Therapist: Will that really help? That's what's called "tit-for-tat."

Manuel: I have a few suggestions for you. I know how you feel because I have a sister who's two years younger. She gets away with doing stuff in my room all the time which I don't like. Usually she gets in trouble. You could chase your sister down the block and then lock the door. You can threaten your parents that you'll run away if they don't finally get a clue.

MN: It emerged, at last: Manuel got to the empathy that the letter-writer was seeking; the helplessness was in the letter. Jacob also had the sense of being on his own with this problem and trying to prove it to his parents: "Won't you believe me?" And then we finally heard from Manuel, "Will you finally believe me?" The boys were now responding to the interaction between the youngster and his parents in this letter. I would have expected this from the girls' group, once again because girls would more stereotypically home in on the "feelings component." Here it's the boys.

GD: I think that boys in this country get stereotyped as aggressive and uncomfortable with feelings. They're viewed as being more apt to hit, call their sisters names. As soon as something happens between a brother and sister, parents may automatically assume that the boy did it if the brother is the older one.

MN: We have to be careful about the tendency to stereotype. It can be so automatic within any culture. I just did it myself.

Manuel: Also, you could lie to her about something. Then when your parents are turned away, you tell her, "*That's* what you get for being mean to me." You could try to make peace with her, but if this is happening all the time, then you need to bug your room like Jacob said. Also, plant little booby traps and fill a bucket full of paint and toss it at her.

Therapist: This sounds like hunters and spies.

MN: You pointed out, with non-judgmental humor, that this was ridiculous and wouldn't lead anywhere. Using humor is very important and it must always be non-judgmental and devoid of sarcasm.

Tyrone: I have two sisters and a brother. One thing you could do is if your sister keeps bugging you, you could take something away and tell her that she won't get it back until she gives you back what she originally took from you. If that doesn't work, just try to make friends with her.

MN: They were looking for justice in a world in which there isn't justice. Instead, there is perceived parental indifference. This group was trying to create fairness between the two siblings because it wasn't going to happen any other way. It's a larger issue than sibling rivalry itself; it is an issue of justice and empathy. These larger issues are often what drive sibling rivalry.

GD: Tyrone, of all the boys, did not see himself as alone. He came from a big family and his mother was exceptionally fair. Her fairness helped Tyrone experience her as empathic and available to him as a resource.

Henry: You have to try to talk to your little sister about it to ask her to stop.

Therapist: A couple of you have talked about making peace.

Duncan: One suggestion is to play her game and annoy her back. Two, try to expose her. Three, make her sign a contract, if you enter my room, then you must dye your hair pink.

GD: The group ended with a mixture of ideas about how to help end the sibling battles. They weren't necessarily good ideas, but the boys were thinking about what might work. Interestingly none of their ideas involved getting parent support, which suggests how alone children in this situation can feel.

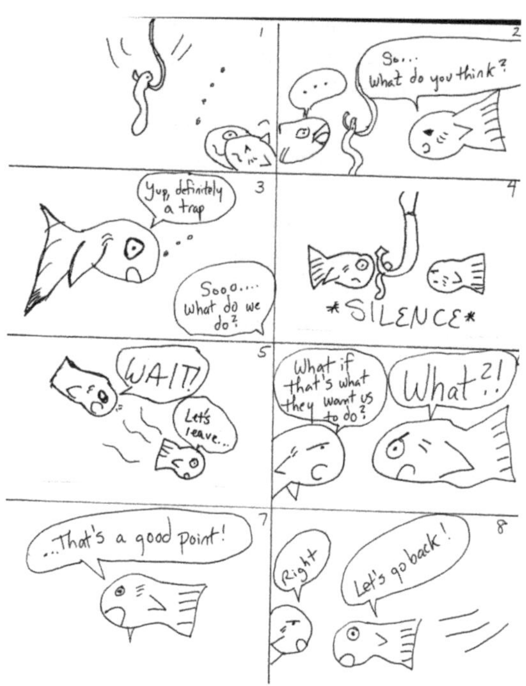

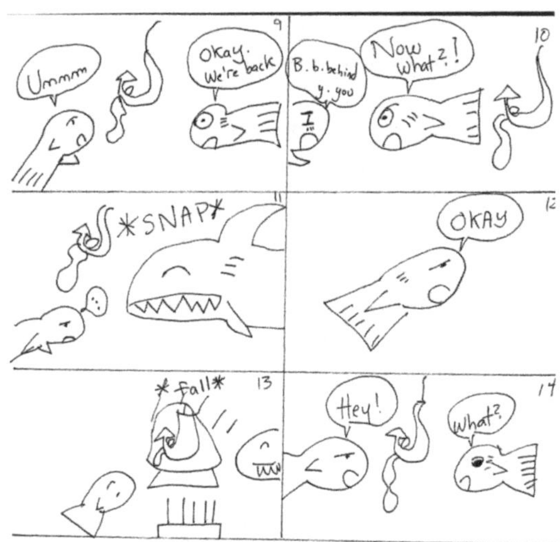
9
Ummmm
Okay. We're back
10
B. b. behind y. you
Now what?!
11
SNAP
12
OKAY
13
fall
14
Hey!
What?

Boys' Group #3

GD: Justin brought a problem of his own to this session and wanted to focus on that rather than the group letter.

Justin: Here's the thing. I have this friend named Ethan. There's a visitor to school named Sam and we were talking about Warhammer™ (a video game). Sam just started school yesterday for the first time and I'm worrying about how to make time with both him and Ethan without alienating either one. Please tell me if you have any solutions.

Tyrone: Simple. Just invite them both to your house. And at school, just make a club and have them both be in your club.

Therapist: Your idea is to try to make both boys be your friends, like a threesome.

Corey: Try to combine Ethan and Sam, but what if they become good friends and they stop being friends with Justin?

Therapist: That's a good question. Justin, are you worried about that?

Justin: No.

Therapist: Good, but it's an important question anyway because things like that can happen.

Leo: I think that you should get all of you enrolled in baseball camp or some other activity together.

MN: That's a good suggestion because Leo was trying to use a very concrete, realistic way of going about dealing with the dilemma. He was looking for something that would help them cohere as a group. It was very specific as well as helpful to the group.

Therapist: That's a good idea. Some activity where they can all have a part.

Oliver: Introduce one to the other and try to find similarities in the three of you. So chances are that you'll become friends. Soon you'll never find one without the other and still have time with them.

Tyrone: If the other plan doesn't work out, split half of recess with one of them and the other half of recess with the other one. I'm still trying to work out how you'd explain that.

GD: Tyrone lacked the capacity to think through the nuances of social interactions and relationships. He had a concrete plan but couldn't work with the interpersonal part.

MN: But Oliver, as opposed to Tyrone, was coming up with something fairly abstract—find similarities so that the three boys in the letter could join each other and have some cohesion. Here was a youngster (Oliver) who was highly depressed, with a history of suicidal ideation. This would suggest a probable chronic feeling of aloneness and possibly a lack of socially supportive people to whom he could turn. And yet he was the boy who found something that really could be done. The process of this group was really helping Justin, and was serving an organizing function for some of the group members.

GD: What these past two groups have shown us are the types of problems that the children were grappling with in their lives. I was always pleased when a child said, "I have a problem for the group" because they were bringing themselves to the group in a highly personal way. Instead of working through displacement, they directly discussed their own selves.

MN: Therefore, the letter became unnecessary.

Suggested Activities

1. Ask the children who has sibling battles at home, who gets blamed for the problems that come up, and what would be fair ways to solve sibling battles. Role-play situations and perhaps generate a videotape on "How to Solve Sibling Battles."
2. Construct a "family sculpture." One child coaches the others to assume the exact gesture and posture of different members of his own family. Then he directs the group members to act out a story about his family.

CHAPTER **16**

Aliens and Earthlings

Which One Am I?

To belong. What can be more important to children? Fitting in with one's peer group is a pivotal experience for late-latency and pre-adolescent children. The ongoing construction of a Self requires the mirroring of peers. By a certain time in a child's life, peers exceed parents in their influence on the course of development. Establishing oneself as an individual requires children to be comfortable with their themselves, their similarities to and their differences from other youngsters. This accomplishment requires the child to feel that her unique personality is enjoyed and accepted by others. When this doesn't occur, she can feel a deep sense of alienation, isolation, and anger. Some children develop a strong sense of self-loathing in the process when they feel different. The following three letters address the issues of belonging to a peer group, and the emotional problems that transpire when children feel alone in their differentness (Box, 1994; Thoits, 1995; Heaney & Israel, 2002). Each letter captures a different aspect of the issues of isolation and alienation.

Dear Kids' Club,

Ever since I was three years old, I have had this one friend, Cory. I am now ten and he is my very best friend. We do all kinds of great stuff together like ride our bikes for hours, make a fort in the woods, and are now setting up a store that we can sell things to kids in the neighborhood. He is really great to be around, but recently I am getting very mad at him. When we were at the pool the other day, he kept playing with some other kids and ignoring me completely. I was getting really mad about it and started pinching him on purpose. This isn't the first time he has done this to me. We were both invited to Raoul's party and Cory was playing ping pong with some other kids. He wouldn't let me in on the match, saying that they already had teams. I was seething inside. I felt so left out and rejected by him. Last year the same thing happened on the playground at least ten times. Doesn't he like me anymore? Should I stay friends with Cory or just try to forget him? Maybe I should do back to him what he is doing to me to get even. I'm really angry about this. What should I do?

Signed,
Louie, the Left Out one
(Louise in girls' version)

GD: I thought this letter would capture issues that many children experience in middle school. I purposely put some aggression in the letter. Although boys are more apt to consider an aggressive response than girls, retaliation of some form is likely to occur when any child feels this way.

MN: Girls are more likely to engage in social manipulation, being verbally critical, even cruel, talking behind the back, or making up stories: "Do you know what she did? Did you see what she was wearing today?" Of course we are using generalizations in this discussion and examples that are "typical" but not exclusive to each gender.

Girls' Group #1

Crystal: This happened to me. I was talking to my friend, Terry, and asked her if she would like to dig a hole with me. She said, "Sure, great!" Then next thing I know I'm over by myself digging the hole and she's off with some other kids. I went over and asked her about it and she said, "Oh, I forgot!"

Therapist: Then what did you do?

Crystal: I went back to digging the hole by myself and I felt really sad.

MN: Crystal was able to begin the group with her initial feelings of anger and then move to her sadness. It looks to me like a defensive transformation of Aggression into Mourning for the perceived lost friendship. It was a good beginning to the group because it brought the affect to the fore.

Therapist: Are you still friends with Terry?

Crystal: Yes. That didn't happen again. But then there was another time that I was digging a hole.

Rosa: You just told that story!

MN: Rosa either wanted to get down to business or to escape the problem. Crystal's way of telling her story avoided the possible fullness of anger that she might have felt. It seems like it was easier for her to start with her anger, briefly touch on it, and then move on to feeling sad. She may have had more to say about angry feelings, but she short-circuited them. She was more comfortable in the world of sadness.

GD: That really did apply to Crystal, who was a very complex child. Here she showed us the complexity in the way she expressed and managed her feelings. It's hard for children to understand dual, or ambivalent, feelings and let themselves have both of these two emotions internally and simultaneously.

Crystal: This is a different time.

GD: Crystal was not going to yield the mike. She needed to tell more of her story.

Crystal: I was digging a hole and the kids that were playing with me went away.

Therapist: Why do you think that happened? Do you think they lost interest in the game or they didn't want to be with you?

GD: I said that because Crystal would do some extremely offensive things to others and be quite unaware of it. I was trying to sensitize her to be more aware. We were along enough in our therapy that I felt that I could bring this issue out in the group—I didn't want the other girls to lose interest in her, but to see that she might have something to offer.

MN: Were you also hoping that the power of peers addressing her behavior (and lack of awareness of it) might have had an impact on her?

GD: I was hoping that peers might give her direct feedback to help her modify her behavior and give her insight. I think it was significant that her story has her digging a hole, just like other children I've worked with who like digging holes: It's a morose, sad, and dark space to go.

MN: It was symbolic. Through her behavior she was "digging a hole for herself," isolating herself from others. It was also a metaphor that might be easy for a therapist to miss because her story was based on a realistic event.

Crystal: I have no idea. Sometimes I have no friends to play with. Like the girl next door to me. I really like her but her mom keeps sending me away, saying that Marissa has homework to do. I feel very lonely sometimes.

Therapist: What about Louise's (the letter-writer's) problem? She has only one friend and feels very left out. Is it a bit like Crystal who also feels lonely and sad?

Rosa: She should try to get another friend so that she doesn't have to rely on just one person all the time. Or she could join a club like Girl Scouts to find more friends.

Therapist: That's a great idea.

MN: Was Rosa trying to "put a period" to this group process? She quite clearly shifted from the world of feelings to the offering of suggestions, very concrete and without any emotions attached.

GD: Yes, I think that was what she was doing. Rosa also could not face the idea that a person might actually contribute to her own plight or cause her own exclusion. She could be very obnoxious and off-putting to the other girls.

MN: We must look not just at the content, but also at the intention of what is being said. "Why is this happening to the group at this exact moment in time?" "What is this group member trying to accomplish by saying what she is saying when she is saying it?" Therefore, we must attend to content, process, and intent of any communication and juggle our multiple awarenesses.

GD: Crystal ended her last statement by talking about being rejected by this girl, Marissa. She had talked about her relationship with Marissa in her individual sessions with me. Apparently Marissa's mother did not want anything to do with Crystal because she was a poisonous kind of child, toxic to other kids. She often played in group and in individual therapy about "being sent away." Crystal's mother also wanted nothing to do with her. It was very sad. That's partly why I pursued Crystal's feelings of loneliness and sadness versus the anger of "digging the hole."

MN: You chose to follow Crystal's sadness-in-the-moment because her sadness was most salient right then. There would always be a time to get back to her anger. Each session is not discrete. Just as each session has its own process, so does the flow of the group across sessions. Groups are usually on a track, a trajectory. They are heading somewhere. We'll always get another chance to say what needs to be said. It's so important that we recognize this and not rush. We must offer our patients something when they are ready to hear it, not out of our own impatience. To put it succinctly: Our patients deserve our patience.

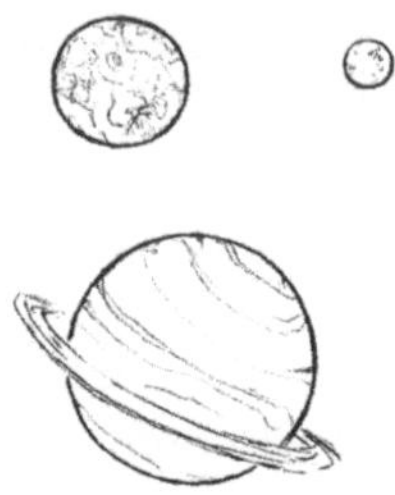

Dear Boys' Club,

I have a very embarrassing problem that really bothers me. I was talking to Georgia about it and she encouraged me to write this letter to you guys. She said that she couldn't tell me any details, but she thought that the boys in your group might have some really good advice for me. She also said that some of you might even have a similar problem and would really understand what I am going through. I'll tell you, just that alone is a major relief to me to know that someone else out there has a similar problem. So here goes.

I am a pretty sensitive guy and now and then I have cried at school. Last year my grandmother died and I was really close to her. In fact, I was closer to her than my own parents. So when she died, it was a major blow to me. This past year my dog got hit by a car and died. When I was at school I broke down and cried a few times just thinking about it. Each time, the kids at school called me "gay." That made me cry even more.

Then there was a time at school this fall, when my friend Sam skidded in the mud on the soccer field and he let out a big yell as he fell. I was just a few feet behind him and was running to make sure he was OK and next thing I knew, I also skidded, but I fell right on top of Sam. When I asked Sam if he was all right, he said he was. And for some reason, the two of us thought it was really funny that we were lying there like a mud sandwich. When we got up, these boys on the team said, "That was so gay."

I am really hurt about being called gay. It happens every day. I have no problem with homosexuals. In fact, my uncle is one and lives with a partner. But I am not gay and I hate being called this if it's not true. Even if it were true, I don't like the way these boys say it to me. I can't imagine what it would feel like to someone who really was gay and had to deal with this all the time. This is getting out of hand, and I don't know what to do. Do any of you have any advice for me?

Signed,
Carlos

GD: This letter evoked a great deal of discussion in the boys' group. Several of them had similar experiences, being called "gay" for being sensitive or having physical contact with peers that was misconstrued. Many of these boys had struggled with the stigma that boys aren't supposed to cry, yet they were faced with the problem of crying easily when bumped, hit, or having their feelings hurt.

MN: Homophobic language begins in full force in Middle School and continues through the first few years of High School. Boys in particular are afraid of feeling vulnerable and our society unfortunately remains homophobic. Thus, when boys call others "gay" for being sensitive, they are expressing their fears of their own vulnerabilities as well as their fears of possibly being "different" in general, whether it is homosexuality, or having an artistic or sensitive temperament, as opposed to an athletic, more outwardly macho disposition.

Boys' Group #2

Kevin: I have a problem called sensory integration, which makes me overly sensitive to touch. I also cry easily when things happen, like not getting picked for teams or that problem I told you about, Matthew, who bumps into me and pushes me in the hallway at school. I have a reputation at school for being the crybaby. I hate it.

GD: Kevin captured some of the impact of sensory integrative dysfunction on peer relationships—how clumsiness and tactile hypersensitivities create social barriers. His response also depicted the anxiety and emotional fragility often experienced by these children.

MN: I'm impressed by Kevin's ability to integrate his sensory integration problems with his emotional sensitivity and with his feelings about it. His response was much more complex than his simple language would suggest. The lesson for therapists is not to be seduced by the simplicity of a youngster's language into thinking that the content is also simple.

Julian: I'm also very sensitive and I cry easily. Last year I cried a lot because my grandmother died. I was closer to her than anyone in the whole world. There were times that I just couldn't control it and would burst out crying in the middle of a class.

MN: It was remarkable that these boys were able to address the issue of their sensitive natures (both emotionally and constitutionally based) so directly. My response, in itself, brings into relief the dangers of a therapist holding preconceived ideas, especially of a group's potential.

Manuel: I know about that. I also cried a lot last year for the same reason. What I did was took breaks to get myself under control.

GD: I was stunned that Manuel could say this to anybody, let alone in a group. He rarely got close to anything personal.

MN: He also spoke in response to the openness of the other boys in the group. He was offering both his feelings and his solution—a nice contribution.

Therapist: Manuel, what did you do?

Manuel: I went to the bathroom to collect myself. Or I'd think of something else.

MN: What do you think happened to Manuel that enabled him to open up in this way?

GD: He developed a sense of instrumentality, a feeling that he could take control of his life, as well as a growing sense of introspection and insight.

Aidan: I wish Ian would stop laughing. It's really disrespectful to Carlos.

GD: The whole time we were talking, Ian was laughing.

Ian: I'm just laughing because of hearing about his uncle being gay. I have no problem with people being gay, homosexual, but hearing it makes me laugh.

GD: Despite his laughter, I could see that he was on the verge of tears.

MN: Being vulnerable struck too close to home. Ian was relying on the use of reaction formation to protect himself from the anxiety of his feelings about being a sensitive child. He was at risk for his defense to fail him and so he reverted to laughing.

Ian: Actually I am just like Carlos. I have been called "gay" a lot at school for similar things, like crying when I'm really frustrated in class, or bumping into kids too much. Julian, didn't you do something just like Carlos this year?

GD: Ian was hyperactive and often bumped into kids just by the nature of who he was. He was a highly emotional and vulnerable child who tended to react to emotionally charged material by either laughing or crying.

MN: Ian wanted to feel joined in his pain. He was, I think rather effectively, asking the kind of question that a group therapist might ask. And Julian responded well to it.

Julian: Yeah. I had that time on the soccer field when I was helping a kid up. I was straddling my legs over him and when I pulled him up, his head was at my crotch and everyone said, "That's so gay." I can't get over it.

GD: That's how the group ended. This letter came at a time when some of the boys in the group were developing a budding interest in girls. Aidan was going to his first dance with a girl the following weekend.

MN: Ian was aware that laughing is a defense. Someone called him on it, and then he was able to explain why he was doing it. He even gave some personal information to explain his behavior. Then, he became aware that his defensive laughing was failing because he came to the verge of tears. He may have looked insensitive at the time, but in fact he was quite sensitive and identified with the general theme of vulnerability. It was good that the therapist didn't criticize Ian for his surface insensitivity—his laughter. It helped Ian state his identification with the letter-writer. The sequence of his response was consistent with suicidal ideation. He internalized his anger and stayed with his sadness—he was on friendlier terms with his sorrow.

GD: It's interesting that you're tuning into Ian's suicidal ideation because we have not spoken about it before. I worried about Ian's vulnerability. In fact, Ian adopted a Goth appearance and often spoke of very dark thoughts.

MN: My process in associating to Ian's material hopefully demonstrates how we can use our therapeutic intuition when we're getting certain data from what a patient or a whole group is expressing. We then have to decide whether to comment or not. This is difficult terrain: I think it's important not to act on pure intuition until we have further validation for ourselves.

GD: I have a mental picture of all these kids because I saw what was happening in the room. You are just hearing their words. Yet, Ian's words alone triggered some intuition in you that something was very wrong. That's what is so compelling about only reading the transcript of the session. You can get distance from the monkey business that boys do in a group and distill the verbal meanings. When a therapist is running a group and is in the thick of it all, she has to hold in mind everything that is going on while containing the group affect and her own reactions to the material being expressed. With Ian, I was resonating to the suicidal ideation, his tenderness, and his pulling away from the group. When Ian was laughing at the beginning of the group, I had to contain my own reaction to it while the boys were talking. I also had to become aware of the process of his response, it's shift within the session. Sometimes it's not just the group that has process, it's also an individual's responses.

MN: You were witnessing, but also experiencing, his laughter, and knew that it was defensive.

GD: Yes, his laughing didn't make me angry at all because I felt that he needed to discharge his emotional tension. I saw that it was irritating Aidan who was experiencing it at face value. Aidan would respond with a moral position, "Stop it already. You're offending the letter-writer." I let the laughter go at first so that it could be discharged. Then I hoped that Ian would collect himself enough to be able to speak about his internal process. I was pleased with his self-disclosure.

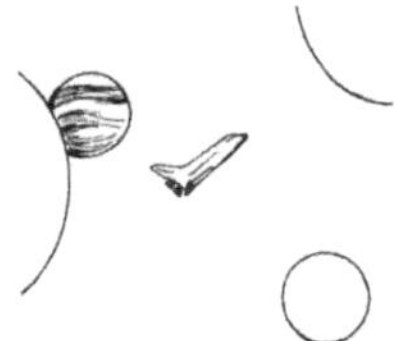

GD: The next letter captures obsessive-compulsive behaviors. One of the boys in the group struggled with this problem, with much pain. Justin's mother was very concerned about his behavior, and this letter was written with him in mind. The ensuing discussion among the authors demonstrates counter-transference and its management.

Dear Kids' Club,

I have a very embarrassing problem and I hope that you will keep this a secret. Whenever I feel stressed, I do certain things in private that make no sense at all, but I have to do them over and over again until I feel just right inside. Like for instance, if my sister is having one of her tantrums, I go into my bedroom and I have this ritual where I rap myself on the head exactly seven times. Then I pinch my forearm up and down seven times. Whenever I go into the bathroom, I have to wash my hands three times, then I touch the black and white tiles back and forth five times. I seem to have this three-five-and-seven number thing going that makes me feel centered. I do this bathroom thing whether I am wrecked out about something or not. Then I have to check and re-check if I have left things in places. I need to go through the room several times to be sure that I have everything that I came with—my backpack, my notebooks, my pen, my Game Boy.

You think that this is the worst of it. Well, it isn't. I also have this thing going in my head with negative thoughts that I get really stuck on. Here's an example. If I raise my hand to answer the teacher and I get the answer wrong, I feel terrible, like I have to punish myself. I say things to myself, "You are a stupid idiot! The most stupid idiot ever alive! You should just go back to preschool and never think about going to school because you are truly a stupid idiot!" Or if my mom gets upset with me that I didn't clean up my stuff from a project I'm working on, then I get going again. I say things in my head over and over like this—"You are the biggest slob in the world. You are like a slug in the gutter. You can't find your stuff. You leave it lying around. You shouldn't even be allowed to have fun because you just make a big mess of everything." I can't stop these negative thoughts.

Does anybody else in your group know about this problem or what you can do to stop? Please help me.

Signed,
Matthew
(Maddie in girl's version)

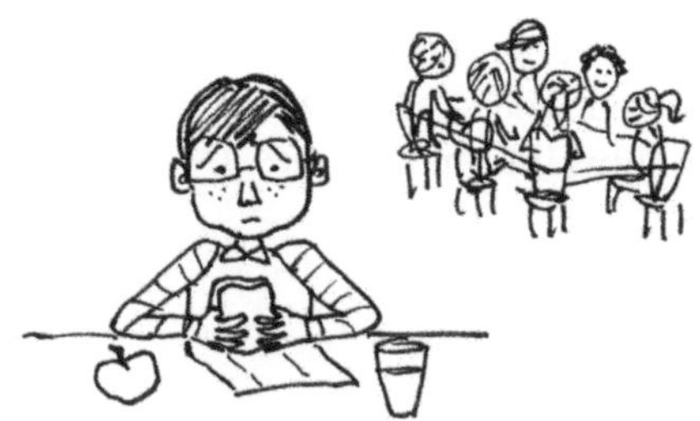

Boys' Group #3

Justin: The brain part, I have this sometimes. When you are checking and rechecking, accept that as a dimension of yourself.

Therapist: A dimension of yourself in what way, Justin?

Justin: Yes, just take it casually. Think of it as nothing really important.

MN: He couldn't deal with the letter-writer's distress about his obsessive-compulsive disorder (OCD). Justin identified with the problem, but he objectified it as something "living" in his brain. That is, it wasn't his problem; it was his brain's problem. This was an excellent example of mind–body separation. It is not a helpful viewpoint because it disintegrates a person into a duality that is really a unity. "Mind" and "Body" can't be separated; mind–body is a single, complex entity. Sometimes I think we have a tendency to forget that.

GD: Yes, Justin did compartmentalize his OCD as a separate aspect of his personality. It certainly would get in the way of his "putting the pieces together" and feeling like a whole, complete, person.

Therapist: So you're saying that when Matthew gets these negative thoughts .... (Justin interrupts.)

Justin: No, I'm talking about the checking and the number thing that he does.

Therapist: Do you have the same thing, Justin?

Justin: I berate myself when things go wrong. Take the checking things as normal.

Therapist: It's just what he does. Do you mean it's just like a habit, like cracking your knuckles?

Justin: Yeah, that's kind of it.

Therapist: Do you have any ideas of what he can do about the thoughts in his head that he can't stop?

MN: The group then inserted itself into the discussion; group process took hold and became more evident.

Jamie: Here's what you do. To get rid of those awful thoughts, play Game Boy all day and watch TV. When you're mom tells you to do an assignment, just do it. When you're eating dinner, here's some advice, get some napkins to clean up your mess.

GD: At the time he said this, Jamie was eating greasy french fries and, without exaggerating, 20 packets of catsup with it. He was covered in it.

Oliver: I have to disagree with the answer you just got from Matthew. I remember that you said that you feel like you're a stupid idiot. If you watch TV and Game Boy all day, you're wasting time to study and chances are, you'll get the answer wrong. I for one would prefer to watch TV and play Game Boy all day, but I don't want to get bad grades. My teachers often tell me that I have a very good academic ability and I just have to learn to use it. Everyone has an academic ability but you have to learn to use it. Maybe that's why my parents won't let me play video games during the week.

MN: I wonder if Oliver was expressing the common problem that some children experience with even well-intentioned helpers: "my teachers tell me I have a very good academic ability and I just have to learn how to use it." He then parroted that advice. But it wasn't really advice; it was just a description. It doesn't lead the child anywhere. We must not fall into this trap of confusing labels with explanations.

Corey: If you get something wrong, you don't have to say you're so stupid. Probably you'll get it right next time. Study a little more and maybe you'll learn it.

GD: Corey also had OCD. Until that moment, he had not contributed to the group discussion for weeks. This was one of the few times he had ever spoken. I was stunned that I got a response from him. It may have been the openness of the other boys that helped him. The main group dynamic in this session was the acceptance of honesty and the safety of self-disclosure.

Therapist: This boy, Matthew, told me that he sometimes worries about the way this voice in his head gets a little out of control. Does this happen to any of you? No?

Oliver: Actually once. It was the beginning of the school year. As many of you may know, many many people called me names and I couldn't tolerate it. A voice in my head said to consider running away or doing some crazy things.

Jamie: That's your conscience gone wild.

Therapist: That's a great point!

Oliver: I was actually thinking that it's your conscience.

MN: I don't understand why Oliver was objecting, or exactly what he was trying to say.

GD: I thought that he was accusing Jamie. It was unusual for Oliver to do something like that. He was a sensitive child and wouldn't hurt others intentionally. I wondered if there was something about this letter that bothered him so much that he had to attack someone.

MN: His response broke the safety that the group had established until then. It sounds as if his fight/flight defense was evoked, laced with some projection. As I think about it, the amount of self-loathing that Oliver felt was probably touching him at a time when he didn't want to be touched. Or the intensity of self-loathing that the letter-writer was expressing was putting Oliver on overload.

Therapist: It's really all in your mind, because you didn't do anything. It has gone wild inside your head.

GD: I wanted to differentiate what's inside versus outside a person's mind.

Jamie: Sometimes the conscience doesn't go wild; sometimes you have messed up and that's when your mind means it. Don't trying eating french fries all day and you'll get messy, so bye.

Oliver: Actually I'm obsessed with Godzilla.

GD: There it was! It took him some time, but then he was not so overloaded and he could talk about something that obsessed him quite a bit. He often talked about Godzilla and his identification with him.

Oliver: The thing that started me to be obsessed with Godzilla, I have trouble with name-calling. When I saw that Godzilla had endured all these fights and not given up, he kind of became an idol for me. A lot of things happened to the actor in the rubber suit playing Godzilla and he doesn't give up. It's not that I'm encouraging you to become a major Godzilla fan, but if you watch a Godzilla movie and put it into consideration, then it may help you put it into perspective. Learn things from watching it.

MN: Although he was talking about Godzilla in a positive way and how Godzilla worked for him, Godzilla was nevertheless a creature that everyone else wanted killed. And justifiably or not (in the movies), Godzilla was still very dangerous, filled with aggression and had the need for revenge.

GD: Godzilla was constructed from the slime of the ocean and came up from the depths as a toxic being.

MN: He was also a mutant creature who was alien, apart from the human world. The humans wanted to rid the world of Godzilla. Oliver used this as a way of organizing his feelings. It troubled me.

GD: I felt during this group, and I'm feeling it now, a deep sense of sadness. I felt flattened and immobilized, unable to speak. I'm noticing that I'm not saying much here either.

MN: I'm a little done in by this material myself and I'm not quite sure what I would have done next. This has such a strong impact on me. When we receive material in a group that is overwhelming to us, it becomes harder for us to continue leading or facilitating the group process. What do we do with the unwanted affect of the client? What do we do when the patient's unwanted affect is also upsetting to us? Do we evoke more process, stay with it, or shift away from it? What do we do when patients' feelings stun us?

GD: If Oliver had said this to me in individual treatment, my response would have been different. In a group, the therapist is containing everyone's affect in the room. When this came flying in at me, I felt devastated internally. I had to put myself on "Pause" because I didn't know how to manage the whole group in that moment other than to shift the group process from discussion of this material to a centering activity that hopefully would have contained, i.e., held onto, the entire group.

MN: How do you mean?

GD: I might have chosen a medium such as clay for them to work on to help center them on an emotional and sensory level. I'd like to bring up something else pertaining to this. Often I will have a dream that will help me to process the material and know the next week what I need to do in the group. It is one of the ways that a therapist might process the unconscious material of a session and make sense of it. For example, I remember once a child constructed a cave from a puppet theatre and blocks in my room. He kept going in and coming out looking scared out of his mind. In my dream I dreamt that there was a skeleton inside the cave. When I awakened, I felt a deep sense of dread that this child was suicidal, which ended up to be true.

MN: It's interesting that you mentioned dreams as a way of processing the material. I sometimes almost will myself to have a dream. "Please dream about this, Marc, and let's see what comes up. Maybe there'll be something here that will help you understand it better."

GD: At times, you have to go to the unconscious to find the real meaning of reality-based reactions and not only symbolism. If Oliver had been in individual therapy, it might have been easier to pick up on this troubling content and follow what he had said the previous week. In a group, that's a bit more difficult to do. You don't have that latitude.

MN: No, you don't, because a therapist would naturally wonder: "if this had such a strong impact on me and I'm the therapist, did it have the same strong effect on the children?" The therapist is stuck on how to respond to Oliver. The next therapeutic task is to assess if the rest of the group is also stuck or if only the therapist's counter-transference is at work. Do you want to go further with the group and this material or not? You have to make that clinical call in the moment.

Suggested Activities

1. Write down on paper what is unique about you that makes you a good friend. Other children in the group can offer feedback about what should be added to the list.
2. Talk about who your friends are, whether it's OK for your friend to have other friends and when you feel left out.
3. Make a group project such as a crayon quilt or a toy or game for a child who is in the hospital. Have shoe boxes, wood pieces, and other found materials available for creations.

References

Box, S. (1994). *Crisis at adolescence.* Northvale, NJ: Jason Aronson.

Heaney, C. A., & Israel, A. (2002). Social networks and social support. In K. Glanz, F. Lewis, & B. Rimer (Eds.), *Health behavior and health education: Theory, research and practice* (3rd ed., pp. 185–209). San Francisco: Jossey-Bass.

Thoits, P. A. (1995). Stress, coping, and social support processes: Where are we? What next? *Journal of Health and Social Behavior,* 1 Suppl., 53–79.

CHAPTER 17
I'm the Best! Right?

"I like myself... don't I?" Self-acceptance should simply occur naturally in the normal course of development. There are two aspects of self-acceptance: (a) liking oneself for who one really is, and (b) wanting to be liked by others for who one really is. When a child dislikes herself, she may manifest it by being a bully or, conversely, by being self-deprecating socially and internalizing the rejection. When others, of any age, dislike a child, that youngster's ability to sustain her acceptance of herself may be compromised. Some children even experience the disapprobation of others as an emotional assault.

This chapter contains two letters. In the first, the child acts superior to others and cultivates the defense of manipulation and rejection of others to validate his position as "the best there is." Underneath his bravado, the child who is truly insecure teases others, name-calls, and insults others in an attempt to perch on an illusionary pedestal.

The second letter uses the insecurities a child might feel when she is adopted and flounders with her personal identity. Often when children are in the age-range of 9–11, they question their roots and wonder how they might be like or not like their biological mother or father. Their search for identity occurs at a time when they are trying to sort out their individual "true self." Their task is to learn how to present themselves to others in ways congruent with who they are. We elected to use adoption as just one example of a child's struggling for identity, and for wanting to be someone worthwhile, because this is a common issue for adopted children (Nemiroff & Annunziata, 2004). However, the general concerns about self-acceptance apply to many children.

Letter #1

Dear Kids' Club,

I'm not really looking for any advice but I thought I'd write to you guys. I'm lucky. I happen to be the coolest kid in my class and really rank status. I'm in the gifted and talented program and I'm smart at just about everything. It's a cinch for me and I don't have to work hard at anything. Smooth sailing it goes! I just wish that I was around more kids like myself instead of those doofuses in my school. I especially hate those Special Ed(ucation) kids across the hall. You should see that one fat kid blubbering down the hall with his mouth gaping open going, "Ahhh, ohhh" and all kinds of weird sounds. Those kids bug me, but the kid who really gets on my nerves is this pest named Thomas. He always follows me around with this look of total adoration on his face. I just want to smash his face in. I tell him to go suck an egg. Sometimes I whack his head with the back of my hand and give him wedgies, but that doesn't seem to stop him. He won't take the hint, so I'm ordering him to do things like he's my slave. Last week I told him to take five dollars out of his mom's wallet and give it to me. He did just like I said, so I'm adding up a list in my head of future deeds. The bottom line is I'd like to unload this brat. He's a real pest. So what should I do?

Signed,
Charlie, the Cool Guy
(Carley in girls' version)

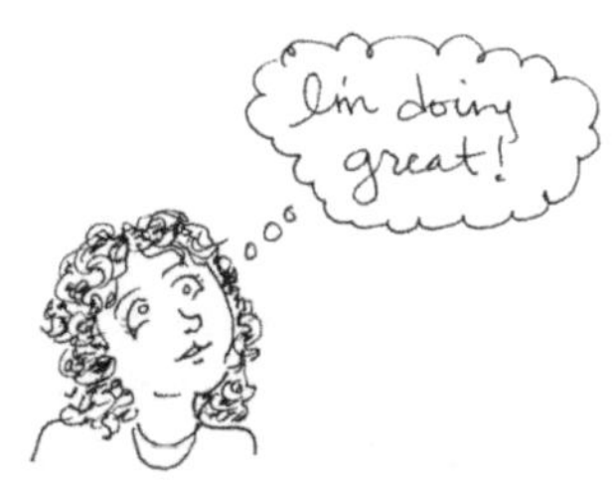

Boys' Group #1

Jacob: You're not asking for advice, but you really need it. That's part of the problem is that you don't realize that you are the problem, not Thomas! You are the real thief for taking five dollars from Thomas' mom.

GD: Jacob surprised me by saying this because he himself was the class clown. Usually he didn't invest energy in meaningful relationships. He acted as if he didn't care. I realized just how much he was putting on a front. Under that façade, he had a truly genuine, softer, side. He needed to feel safe enough to let that part of himself emerge.

Duncan: There was a kid who bumped into this other kid at my school, pushing him down to the floor because he followed him around all the time. It really bugged him, but the follower didn't get the message even after he was knocked around.

MN: Duncan was expressing futility. I don't know if he was simply resonating to the letter or if he was trying to figure out where the responsibility lay. It sounds like Duncan was not responding to Jacob, but was speaking instead about the letter, ignoring what Jacob had just said. Duncan disrupted the group process that had begun.

GD: Duncan's Asperger's would have led him to associate to a concrete event rather than respond to Jacob's insight about the letter-writer. Jacob was more able to put the problem in an abstract, ethical, framework.

Tyrone: If this kid would take this advice, it would help. Find other ways to make him go away. Pretend he's not there. Ignore him and he'll stop following you. Just don't bully him. That's mean.

GD: Tyrone was trying to help the letter-writer out, giving specific advice to get rid of this pest rather than simply saying, "Stop bullying him." The group wasn't empathizing with the Special Ed child who was shadowing the letter-writer so annoyingly.

MN: The group wasn't attending to the victimized child in the letter. This letter is really about exploitation in relationships, and how a child who doesn't like himself can turn into an exploiter. Duncan's social misreading contributed to his response. This is an interesting process when you consider what Tyrone had said. It was Tyrone who had introduced the moral issue.

Manuel: Girls call me a loser all the time at school. One girl in particular does it. I try to ignore her and think about other things. I know I'll be going to the Science Convention and get an A+ though, and she'll get the C. The only problem is so far she is also getting A's.

GD: Manuel was not the type of Special Ed child who was a follower, but he had been known to do really problematic things, such as behaving as if he were stalking another child. He might adore someone and follow him relentlessly until that youngster would complain to the principal. Manuel liked to go to science-fiction conventions. He often spoke extensively about this and didn't understand that the other boys had had enough. He clearly didn't read the cues that he was starting to be annoying. His "stalking" behavior usually involved girls whom he admired.

MN: Did he understand the inappropriateness of his behavior? Was he capable of becoming attuned to the irritation of the other child? Was there any malice? There doesn't really seem to be.

GD: Manuel was actually very sweet and wouldn't become overly focused on the other child out of malice. His thinking and behavior had more of an obsessive-compulsive flavor. He would develop a crush on a girl, misread the social cues, and not know what to do next.

MN: Manuel's comments in the group raise an important therapeutic issue. We have here a youngster who <u>looked as if</u> he might have been frightening because of his behavior (the "stalking"), when in fact he really just cared about another person and couldn't read the social cue: "stay away." He was certainly not a dangerous child; he was more what I would call a "dys-cued" child. A therapeutic group has the potential to teach him a lot about social cues. Youngsters with such problems as Manuel's are sometimes seen as inappropriate for group therapy when in fact group treatment, with well-matched members, sometimes is the treatment of choice.

GD: Manuel participated in group psychotherapy for several years and did make progress in reading social cues, but this problem of "stalking" children whom he admired continued to be a problem. When I saw him for individual treatment, we finally made headway by teaching him explicit strategies as soon as he became alert to the fact that he was obsessing over another child. The real work lay in my helping him to feel more secure with who he was so that he was less reliant on using others to define himself.

Duncan: I'm a loser when it comes to running but when it comes to video games I'm a winner.

MN: Duncan resonated to the issue of victimization—"I'm the loser," but tried to find a way to end this thought with a situation in which he would be a winner. His mentioning both of these social positions, the winner and the loser, in one unbroken sentence demonstrated his anxiety. He moved from the intolerable "being a loser," to the desirable "being a winner." He was talking about how often he thought of himself as a loser. His pain was exposed in his pressured language—that unstoppable sentence.

GD: Looking between the run-on lines, he made a lovely connection to the letter-writer. He was trying to tell Charlie that there are two sides of the coin—the struggles that Special Ed children might experience when they aren't so competent.

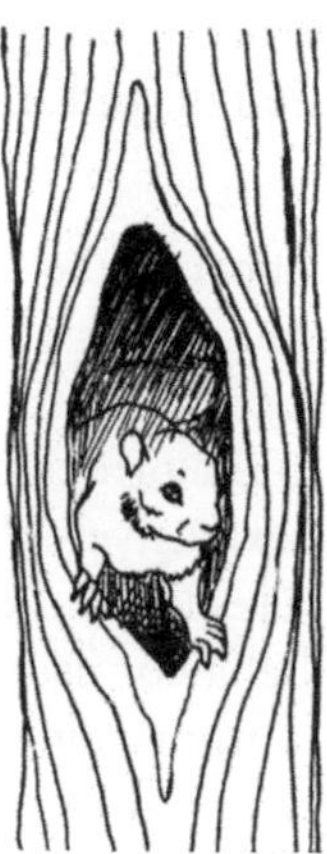

Letter #2: Concerns about Being Adopted and Self-Acceptance

GD: This letter is about being adopted. There are a high number of adopted children in my groups. During the time that I was running these particular groups, more of the girls had been adopted than the boys. This will be apparent in each group's responses to the following letter. It depicts many of the concerns that adopted girls have expressed to me.

MN: We have selected one group in particular because the girls' responses touch on the important issues and also raise salient therapeutic considerations.

Dear Kids' Club,

I am adopted. When I was 3 months old, my biological mom gave me up for adoption. I am not sure the reason why, but I think that it is because my mom had a big problem with drinking and had some nasty boyfriends who yelled a lot. I was actually put in a foster home for a month before my adoptive parents found out about me and gave me a home.

My adoptive family is really nice. My mom and dad give me a lot of attention and take me to a lot of good activities like gymnastics (soccer), guitar lessons, and Girl(Boy) Scouts. I also like my older sister who is in high school. She's really nice to me, too. The only bad thing about my adoptive family is that my mom and I don't always see eye to eye about things and we fight about stuff like when I want to buy a new toy, or I want to wear a certain outfit and she disagrees, or I don't feel like working on my homework right then.

So what is the problem? Two things. I am really ashamed about being adopted. I don't want any of my friends to know about my real mom because it is a total embarrassment. They might think that I will end up a drunk like she was or be violent because I think she was that way too. My friends might think that I will be a bad influence on them, like a poison. But besides that, I am very hurt that my biological mom gave me away. I feel so rejected by her and think that maybe if I found her, I could talk to her and find out what really happened. Did she ever really love me? And why did she give me up if she did love me? I sometimes worry that I'm not lovable and that my adoptive family just feels sorry for me, like I'm a charity case and that that's the only reason why I'm here.

I'm not sure what advice I am looking for. Is anybody in your group adopted and how do they feel? Do they want to know about their real mom or dad? Do they worry about being rejected and not loved by their adoptive family? Also, are they ashamed about this and keep it a big secret? Please tell me.

Signed,
Julie
(James in boys' version)

GD: As I read this letter now, I realize that it's pretty sophisticated for a child to write.

MN: Still, it's heart-wrenching and brings up many of the issues of adopted children.

Girls' Group #3

Deborah: You don't know that your mom was a drunk because no one told you that. Most parents give their child away because they do love them and they can't care for them and they want them to be in a better home. Or maybe they're homeless or something and they can't care for them. That is loving them and it's not giving them away because they don't love them. She probably wasn't a drunk.

GD: While Deborah was talking, Alexis, a Russian adoptee, sat there looking very shut-down. The story of the letter-writer was so close to Alexis's reality that she could have written this letter herself.

MN: I wonder if, within the therapeutic moment, Alexis was truly shut-down and, therefore, nothing was coming in or was she being very quiet while actually taking it all in. If it was the latter, she was indeed participating in a positive group process and many of the girls in the group would have been aware of it. If it was the former, her being shut-down could have had a negative effect on how the group proceeded. "Diagnosing the Silence" is a particularly difficult therapeutic skill.

Gillian: When you're adopted it feels kind of sad because I was never adopted, thank God. If you were adopted, then you might not get the same privileges. You still can live a happy life with your adoptive parents. They will still love you. Tell your mom and dad if you are not happy though.

MN: Gillian was speaking as if an adopted child is loved but not as much as a biological child. She was making it sound as if an adopted child would be better off than she was before, but nevertheless remain a "second-class citizen" and would be, in a sense, "damaged." Biological children, too, often feel like "second-class citizens," particularly when they are engaged in intense sibling rivalry. We really need to say here that feeling like a "second-class citizen" is not the exclusive domain of the adopted child. It would be helpful if some adopted children could understand this.

GD: I think that Gillian viewed herself in that way because she had cerebral palsy. She often brought this up in her individual therapy sessions. It's like you were just saying: it isn't only adopted children who feel that there is something wrong with them. Gillian's example is of having a physical condition, but lots of youngsters who don't have physical conditions, and who are not adopted, share these same feelings and worries about whether they are worthy or not.

MN: Gillian identified with the letter-writer as being "not as good as," or not as intact at core, as other children. She seemed to make the connection that being adopted can feel like being damaged.

GD: Still, we mustn't forget that she still felt that adoptive parents would always love their adopted children: This was the blessing that her parents had given her.

Deborah: My friend was adopted from China when she was one year old. Kids sometimes say to her, "You're adopted" or "You're Chinese." I don't think it bothers her all that much. Also, in China there is a law that you can only have one child. So you have to give up the child whether you want to or not.

MN: Deborah was clearly trying to work with the rejection issue and came up with a justification for it. She was troubled by the idea of a child not being wanted. The group was working quite well with the difficult issues of rejection, damage, and acceptance.

Ashley: One of my cousins is adopted. She fights a lot with her mom, then in school she says something and people ask her questions. They don't think that it makes her bad. When she gets annoyed about it she says, "Why are you asking questions about my mom?" Then people stop. They don't care; they just think it's interesting. It's a curiosity. We don't know so many people from other countries.

Alexis: I was adopted from Russia. I've been sharing it and people don't laugh at me.

GD: Ashley's comment helped to resurrect Alexis. I was pleased that she stepped forward to speak about herself. I knew that she was deeply troubled about her adoption, so I invited her to respond further.

MN: It's a nice example of a young group member making the key therapeutic comment. I love it when those moments occur in group, when the therapist becomes extraneous.

Therapist: Have you ever experienced any of the things that this girl wrote about?

Alexis: No.

Therapist: Do you ever fight with your mom, girls? That happens with a lot of girls whether they're adopted or not.

MN: I'm so glad that you generalized your comment. It brought the commonality of feelings of self-acceptance and worthiness out in the open and made it clear that it applies to everyone.

GD: I decided to end the session with a comment about the letter-writer's relationship with her own mother. The sad thing about Alexis was that she had just been sent away to a residential school. She wasn't told this information until just a few weeks before it happened. Her parents couldn't control her at home. Two weeks before, her mother called me to tell me that Alexis was having a lot of behavioral problems at the residential school. "She's acting up! They can't control her! What will we do now? She can't come home and we can't have her in our home. We can't handle this child." This was heart-wrenching, and of course Alexis experience the rejection as profound. It's quite possible that Alexis set it up to act-out at the school to see if her parents loved her enough to take her back again.

MN: It was, I believe, a repetition compulsion. The fantasy was probably that her birth mom didn't want her, and Alexis tested her adoptive family to see if they would give her up as well. She was acting out her underlying question of her own worth, her "keepability," and unconsciously repeating her fantasy of what originally happened to her. I think we can extrapolate from her theory that she was adopted because there was something inherently defective about her. By the time she was in group, she was testing her adoptive parents: "What if I do this; will you still keep me?" "And if I do something <u>this</u> bad, will you throw me out?" "Will you unadopt me?"

GD: This pattern is very common with children who come from backgrounds like these adopted girls. When a child is dealt a bad deck developmentally and has a host of learning disabilities combined with mood disorder, she is likely to struggle in any family, whether she is adopted or not. The sad part of the story is that sometimes a residential placement is the only solution when a child is so out-of-control.

MN: This letter is laden with emotion and addressed to a group in which half of the girls were adopted. It should have led to a great deal of conversation and self-disclosure. In a way, this letter failed. Why is that so? This is a very rich letter, but the group's response to it was quite defended. We always try to ask ourselves: "what happened?"

GD: There are several letters in this book that I was surprised did not hit the mark and elicit the kind of conversational discourse and process that many of the other letters did. I think this letter depicted emotions in too raw or pure a form. Perhaps if I had wrapped the letter-writer's concerns in more of a defensive tone or with more bewilderment, it might have worked better. The letter-writer was really putting the rejection right out there. It was too raw and the group needed to back away.

MN: So the girls were not able to utilize their defenses against their anxiety effectively enough to respond to the letter. They were confronted with too much emotionality in the letter. The best they could do in a situation like that was a variation of a shut-down, flight rather than fight. They almost shut the door on you. If we can maintain our own self-acceptance, we can learn from this as therapists. The children needed their more adaptive defenses in order to function and talk about themselves.

GD: In writing this letter, I assumed that it, in itself, was a displacement, but I peeled away too much and did not consider the defensive position that these kids needed in order to respond to the topic. This lesson teaches us how to write a letter!

MN: It also brings up what kind of facilitating comments a therapist might make in a group. It's so important to be as careful as possible when children move into emotional territory that is difficult, and to let them know that we respect their defensive space.

GD: The techniques that I often used in group to facilitate children might have been normalizing comments such as "many children feel this way," self-disclosure with a pertinent example, or validation of the distress, anxiety, or feeling tone that a group experiences in that moment. When these strategies failed to yield the desired result, I resorted to a non-verbal medium or activities that grounded the children and focused the group process. Sometimes, after the children had distanced from the material in the letter and were absorbed in their activity, they became able to talk about or express non-verbally the residual feelings that were stirred up by the letter.

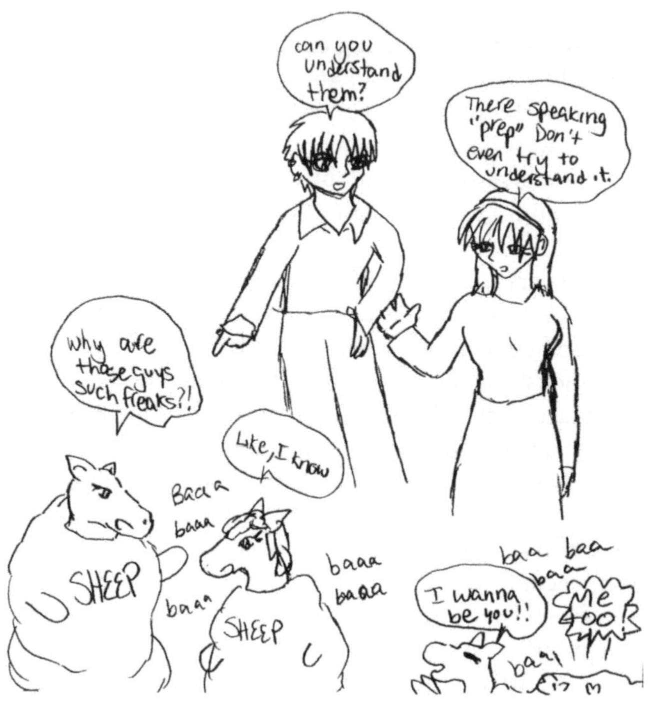
can you understand them?
There speaking "prep" Don't even try to understand it.
why are these guys such freaks?!
Like, I know
Baa a
baaa
SHEEP
baaa
SHEEP
baaa
baaa
baa baa
baa
I wanna be you!!
Me too!
baa

Suggested Activities

1. Each child picks a character they would like to be in a story. Develop what and who the character is—what they look like, how old they are, what they like to do, what they don't like to do, and what their attributes are. The children may fill out a sheet about their character, including things like what makes your character happy? Sad? Angry? Have each child draw a picture of their character. This can be made into a paper doll.
2. Develop a group story based on the characters. Have children draw scenery for the backdrop, then make a show with their paper doll characters.

Reference

Nemiroff, M., & Annunziata, J. (2004). *All about adoption: How families are made and how kids feel about it*. Washington, DC: Magination Press.

CHAPTER **18**

Impulsivity vs. Social Inhibition

"I'm too Scared to Speak" vs. "I Couldn't Help Myself"

Social Inhibition

Many children with social problems experience difficulties with pragmatic language. They find themselves verbally at sea, not knowing what to say to other children, and struggling with the basics of conversational discourse. Children with problems in the use of pragmatic language often don't get past the very basics of communication. Verbal dysfunction precludes the development of intimacy in relationships. The conversation of such youngsters tends to be sparse and superficial because they have not developed the capacity to verbally express a higher-level discussion of thoughts or feelings. In addition, a child may have memory deficits that cause him to forget what he wanted to say, or he may have poor gestural communication and fail to make good eye contact, or provide relevant facial or gestural feedback to others. Other children may perceive them as aloof or disinterested.

A vicious cycle then develops such that the child never gets the social feedback he so desperately needs. In addition, children with pragmatic language deficits often do not read and process the gestural and facial cues of others. They confuse or misinterpret the social meanings and communicative intentions of others. Children with these kinds of difficulties often live with a high degree of anxiety about approaching others, not knowing what to say or do to create conversation (Adams, Green, Gilchrist, & Cox, 2002; Gillot, Furniss, & Walter, 2001; Towbin, Pradella, Gorrindo, Pine, & Leibenluft, 2005). The current letter addresses what such difficulties are like.

Dear Kids' Club,

It is hard for me to write this letter because I don't know how to explain my problems. I can never think of anything to say to kids. My mind is a complete blank. They can be talking to me and the next thing I know, they just walk away. I don't even know what happened. I didn't see it coming. When someone asks me a question, I sometimes forget what I wanted to say. It's like the idea flew out of my head. The funny thing is that sometimes I think of what I wanted to say hours later. I might even wake up with it in my head. My mom is always saying, "Go over to that kid and say hi. Start a conversation." She doesn't know how hard that is for me. I go over and stand there, looking around at the trees, or my shoes, or other things, then I look at the kid. He must know how nervous I am. My mom says, "Start a conversation." But what about? I have no idea. So what should I do?

Signed,
Spencer, the Shy Guy
(Stephanie in girl's version)

GD: I wanted to capture in this letter what it is like for children who have delays in pragmatic language and who also experience social anxiety when confronted with the task of conversation.

MN: The letter also addresses the confusion these children often feel. Difficulties with pragmatic language make social interaction so hard and anxiety-inducing. The mother is benign, urging the child to start a conversation, but the youngster doesn't know how to do it. What is the next step? Very often children get taught the first sentence: How do you start a conversation, but really what they have trouble with is: what do you say next? How do you maintain the conversational flow?

GD: Problems with pragmatic language are often why children attend social skills groups. Difficulties with conversational discourse can tie a child up in anxious knots. Oftentimes they are more comfortable interacting non-verbally, but the reality is that by the time they reach latency age and middle school, their peers are more competent interacting verbally and have left them behind. These youngsters get left in the dust, missing out on vital interactions with their peers, and precluding further possibilities for learning necessary communication skills with their age-mates.

Girl's Group #3

Alexis: I started off like you, and I used to be really really shy and at school I wouldn't talk to anybody, and at recess I would be out on a field with the woods all around. Close by was this pond and I would always be by the pond, out of people's sight. That way they couldn't see me. There I would feel relaxed, but after a while I started to feel lonely. Then I needed somebody to play with so I made friends with this boy named Lee. We went to the pond together and we caught the frogs and toads and tadpoles and that kind of stuff. Then I became very social. Now I'm at a new school and I have a lot of friends. At my other school I didn't have friends though, except one and that was Lee. Maybe if you're alone for some time and have nobody to talk to. Maybe this could help you. You could look for somebody to talk to.

Therapist: It's great advice. Alexis. What you brought up is that you played with Lee in more action kinds of play: looking for tadpoles and not using words very much. Maybe that was the bridge to talking, finding something to do where words weren't so important.

MN: Alexis's way of addressing this was poetic. It was wistful and she was trying to be helpful as well. She was also aware that her own shift was a process. Instead of some direct advice to the letter-writer, she said, in effect, "This took me some time. This is what I started to do, and then I started to feel this way, and then I was able to do this." There was maturity in her understanding. Other youngsters in the group could learn from this. These kinds of problems take some time to overcome. There's an arc toward a solution.

GD: I was really taken aback, because Alexis was a Russian adoptee who had few attachments to anyone. Yet when given the structure of a letter to respond to, she could describe herself as feeling lonely. She was talking about the process of how she could become a social being who could learn to seek intimacy with others.

MN: She was also talking about feeling safe with the enclosing woods all around her. She evoked a mother image: the pond. Then she spoke of tadpoles. They are creatures that transform and grow. So even her symbolism showed the process of moving away from being close to home, that is, starting with one "form," and then transforming into another, making her way in the world around her. It was lovely how she used these symbols.

GD: This letter spoke to her in a powerful way. We know this by the level of her response.

Alexis: Everyone was teasing me and saying that I was friendly with a boy.

Deborah: If you're going to talk to people you should know that a lot of people are shy and they're hoping the other person is going to say something. They want the other person to break the ice. If you do, they'll feel much better because you're in control of the conversation. Pretty soon they'll be starting conversations with you. You shouldn't be afraid to say it.

MN: That was similar advice to the mother in the letter: "Start a conversation." It wasn't bad advice, but it didn't really help. There was also an element of control in it: "you're in control of the conversation." Feeling in control of the conversation would provide a defensive, if illusory, sense of comfort. Youngsters like this need "how to" help.

GD: Deborah had Asperger's syndrome and her comment may have represented her way of working out a conversation in advance. Rote learning about social situations can be very helpful to youngsters who have Asperger's.

Gillian: You should say, "Hey, Mom. I'm feeling really shy and angry because no one likes to hear my ideas. Or they like my ideas but not me. Mom, you don't really get it, and you're supposed to help me. If you do that, that would really help me." Think about talking to your mom and dad instead of walking away from this.

Therapist: That's good. Do you have firsthand experience with this?

GD: I was trying to help the group address the shyness that the letter-writer was experiencing and the feeling that no one liked to hear what she might have been thinking or feeling.

MN: Gillian was offering advice that was more instrumental: "say more about what you need to the people who could help." She was trying to help the letter-writer find ways to feel less victimized by her disability within a social situation.

Gillian: Yeah. When I was younger, I had no friends, then I met this cute boy and we became friends. That was in fifth grade. He is such a sweet boy. Now I'm a big chatterbox.

Elizabeth: If you're not sure what to say, think about what you want to say before you go up to the person. Say in your mind what you want to talk about. This is how I'm going to start the conversation.

GD: Elizabeth was just like the child in this letter. She needed to plan in advance what to say in any conversation. Unfortunately, by the time she got the nerve to speak up after formulating what she wanted to say, the conversation had galloped off in another direction. Elizabeth would miss her opening, and end up being overlooked and not reinforced for contributing to the conversation.

Therapist: That's a great idea—plan ahead.

Ashley: I'm kind of shy with meeting people. What helps is bringing up topics that the person is interested in. Like I know a person who is interested in art and she likes to talk about that. It's not a good idea to bring up topics that are one-word answers. Then it's kind of awkward because once you ask the question, then there's nothing to talk about. It's a good idea to bring up topics that can lead to more things to talk about.

GD: I had just met with Ashley the week before in an individual therapy session and we had come up with these ideas. She demonstrated in her comment that she was in the process of internalizing these strategies.

MN: From a process framework, the girls were in fact having a conversation with each other. They were talking to the letter-writer and to you, but they were also really listening to each other and responding to each other at quite some length. It would have been interesting to label that, to know what it's like to have a conversation with one another. "You girls just had a conversation." They would have been told that they had just experienced some ease with the very problem that they were discussing.

GD: That would have been a good way to end the group.

Social Impulsivity

The inability to control oneself—impulsivity—is a problem of self-regulation that many children with attention-deficit hyperactivity disorder (ADHD) experience. In its way, it presents social problems as important as shyness does: sometimes the "real person" underneath gets overlooked because of the manifest symptomatology. It is common for children with ADHD to do impulsive, outrageous things, acting before thinking. After an impulsive act, these children often experience remorse or embarrassment, and are painfully aware that they used poor social judgment. The ability to "put the brakes on" before acting out, couples with the ability to disrupt an impulsive action mid-stream, is lacking (Barkley, 1997; Brown, 2005).

> *Dear Kids' Club,*
>
> Let me start this out with some important information about me. I am a really nice kid and everyone likes me, except for my big sister who is a pain in the neck. My problem is that I happen to do things on sheer impulse. I get the idea in my head, and next thing I know, I do it! I was looking at this kid's ear and thinking how weird it looked. The ear lobes were really big and floppy looking, like an elephant's. Next thing I know, I'm wiggling them! Funny, eh? Here's another example. I love to use my sister's

Game Boy and sneak into her room and steal it when I get the impulse. No matter how much I say to myself, “Don’t do it! Don’t do it!” I just can’t control myself and next thing I know, there I am with her Game Boy in my hands. I do the same thing with my mom’s secret chocolate stash. I raid that regularly. She keeps changing her hiding place but I outsmart her. Some of the things I do are harmless. What’s wiggling a kid’s ear? But sometimes the things I do aren’t so harmless! Like the other day, I was sick and tired of this kid talking and talking and talking. He wouldn’t shut up! So I just put my hand right over his mouth and held it there. Boy, did that get me in trouble. It was like a federal offense. They sent me home from school that day. What would you recommend for me about my “Impulse Problem?”

Signed,
Peter, the Impulsive
(Inez in girls’ version)

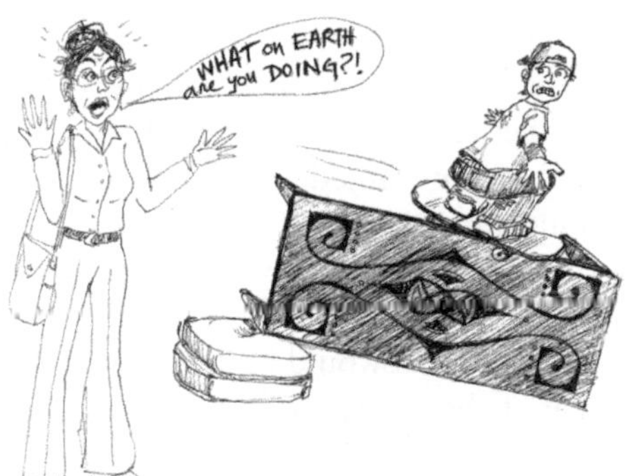

Girls’ Group #1

Rosa: Here’s my advice. Just don’t do these things. You have to ask for the chocolates and stay away from your sister’s Game Boy. And you should be nice to hear things from that kid.

Therapist: You mean for her to let him talk to her? But it was annoying to her. She couldn’t stand it anymore.

Rosa: Maybe you should buy some earplugs. Maybe that would help.

Therapist: That’s an idea. Just ignore him or put earplugs in. Let me ask you this. Does anybody in here have this kind of problem of doing things they shouldn’t?

Crystal: Definitely. I have this friend and he talks up a storm and when I ask him to be quiet, he’ll say, “What?” Then I ask him, “Could you please be quiet?” And he keeps on talking. But then a minute after, the teacher asks him to be quiet, like we’re onto the next thing. When she asks him to be quiet, he’s quiet, but when I ask him to be quiet, he isn’t. He likes the teacher better than me and he listens to her.

Therapist: Crystal, do you ever do things that you shouldn’t do?

Crystal: Yeah.

Therapist: That’s what Inez is saying. She wants to stop doing these things but she can’t.

Crystal: Sometimes I sneak into my mom’s room and take her binoculars. Last time I did it a piece broke off.

Therapist: You know that you shouldn’t have been doing that, but you did it anyway.

Crystal: Yes, I did it anyway. Then she said, "Did you break my binoculars?" And I'm like, "What did you ask?" She said, "Did you break my binoculars?" Then I said, "Say that again." She said it again. "Please leave a message after the beep and I'll get back to you."

Therapist: Who said that, you did?

Crystal: Yeah.

Therapist: I guess that's one solution. Become an answering machine.

Crystal: She asked me one more time and I said, "Yes, I confess. I did. I'm sorry." They're like the real expensive kind. The big, heavy black kind.

Therapist: What if tonight you get the urge to take those binoculars? What will you do?

GD: I wanted to evoke the particular moment when she felt the impulsive urge.

MN: There was a therapeutic dilemma and you had to make a choice. With the binoculars, was there some emotional or literal voyeurism? I don't mean in the truly perverse sense, but in the sense of wanting to see or know? With binoculars you have some distancing in looking at others. You're farther away but you can see up close, often without other people knowing that you're looking. The specific therapeutic choice was whether you preferred to stress the emotional meaning of the symbolism or whether you wanted to stay on the purely group-level response to this letter and its meaning. Do you follow Crystal's apparently individual symbolic meanings that were triggered by the letter or do you stay on the manifest group-level importance of the topic at hand? Was Crystal speaking for the group or not? Having a sense of that would be a guide for the therapist's decision.

GD: Here's another side of the story. I was intrigued when Crystal brought up the binoculars. Her mother was a peculiar woman who looked rather cloistered and puritanical. When she sat in our waiting room, I frequently found her looking at ads in magazines for Viagra or lingerie. Sometimes she would make very inappropriate remarks to me about my appearance. If I had on an outfit that she thought was cute, she might say to me, "Ooooh! I bet your husband likes that!" There was something quite odd, even unsettling, about it. Crystal's father and mother were a disengaged couple. He would go out tango dancing and leave her at home. There was something voyeuristic about her mother that was sexualized. I chose not to pursue this material in the group context. I thought to myself: "I'm not going there with the binoculars—what one sees with them."

MN: You respected your own boundaries and counter-transference, which was a good idea. A therapist must feel safe, just as a patient should, within the therapeutic situation. You would have had to move into territory that didn't feel good to you, and so you didn't. Therefore, it became very important not to pursue the binoculars' issue.

GD: If I had been working with Crystal in an individual session and this material emerged, I would have explored it, but not in a group setting because I felt that it was too close to something that was happening in Crystal's family life. I did not want to uncover this in the group so that I could protect her.

MN: You kept Crystal and yourself safe. If you had pursued this, it would have put the group in the position of being voyeurs as well. Your own counter-transference helped contain this.

Crystal: I'll just say, "Why don't we go do something else" to myself? I really have been interested in them lately. Last time I looked for them, I thought they were in the living room closet but they're in my mom's closet and I can't reach up there. It's too high.

Therapist: Do you think your mom would let you have them if you asked?
Crystal: She'll probably say, "The last time you had them you broke them." I'll say, "I won't do it this time."
Therapist: Maybe if you get her trust back, she'll agree to let you borrow them.

MN: Rather than follow the meanings and the personal troubles we just talked about, you stayed with the literal binoculars. Interestingly, the rest of the group dropped out of this discussion. "The group" had become a conversation between you and Crystal. I think that the group had become aware that this was uncomfortable, dangerous ground and therefore not safe.
GD: It's important for a group therapist to pay attention to when the process becomes dyadic versus group-level. When you have a dyad, you know you've lost the group. That's when it's important to shift gears and make a transition to an activity that facilitates group interaction. This particular group responded best when I organized group art projects. I usually chose ones that allowed each child to do a solo project that could be merged together into a group activity. As a therapist, it feels like working with puzzle pieces in order to find a way to construct a whole from the parts.

Suggested Activities

1. Using the characters and scenery developed in the previous chapter, videotape a story. For children who need help with this, the therapist may need to prompt different aspects of the story line. How will it begin? What interesting, puzzling, adventurous, strange, disastrous events happen in this story? What might the characters be feeling when these things occur? How to make a story so that all the characters get a major role? How will the story end? Will it be a happy ending, or one that leaves the audience scratching their heads wondering what is the next episode?
2. Take two children from the group into another room and videotape a conversation about an interesting topic. The group leader may offer them several topics to pick from. For example, one child may be a parent reprimanding a child for not coming home after an event. Or the leader may prompt the children to pretend they are two siblings fighting over who gets to sit in the front seat of the van. Or the children can play act one telling the other that his pet guinea pig just died. Videotape a range of scenes with different combinations of children. Play the videotape with the sound off for the rest of the group and ask the children to figure out what the actors were feeling or thinking and to guess what they might have been talking about.

References

Adams, C., Green, J., Gilchrist, A., & Cox, A. (2002). Conversational behaviour of children with Asperger syndrome and conduct disorder. *Journal of Child Psychology and Psychiatry, 43*, 679–690.
Barkley, R. A. (1997). *ADHD and the nature of self-control.* New York: Guilford Press.
Brown, T. E. (2005). *Attention deficit disorder: The unfocused mind in children and adults*. San Antonio, TX: Harcourt.
Gillot, A., Furniss, F., & Walter, A. (2001). Anxiety in high-functioning children with autism. *Autism, 5*, 277–286.
Towbin, K., Pradella, A., Gorrindo, T., Pine, D., & Leibenluft, E. (2005). Autism spectrum traits in children with mood and anxiety disorders. *Journal of Child and Adolescent Psychopharmacology, 15*, 452–464.

PART III
Emotional Regulation

Children often are unaware of what they are feeling, even though their behavior makes it quite clear to those around them. Emotional regulation is an important developmental achievement (DeGangi, 2000; Greenspan, 2003). The ability to accomplish this is sometimes compromised in children with constitutionally based regulatory problems. These youngsters require modifications to a more typical therapeutic approach.

Part III demonstrates how children with regulatory problems work with the narrative therapy letters to learn to identify and understand their emotions. These letters focus on internal distress, anger, impulsivity, and frustration in everyday life. They were written with the additional goal of helping children gain insight and control of such feelings as sadness, embarrassment, guilt, and anxiety.

CHAPTER 19
"Feeling Blue"

Depression in children manifests itself in several ways. One child may become sullen and withdrawn and may experience an overwhelming sense of sadness. Another child might become passive and withdraw from things that used to give him pleasure. He may withdraw from his friends and begin to say disparaging things about himself, feeling that he is stupid or incompetent. Other depressed children manifest it in a different way. They become intense, irritable, and highly reactive with outbursts of anger and negativity. In other cases, youngsters show more variability of mood with fluctuations between happy and excitable states to sadness or defiance. This latter pattern is sometimes characteristic of children with bipolar depression (Geller & DelBello, 2003; Greenspan & Glovinsky, 2002).

There are three letters in this chapter. Children in two different groups wrote two of them. Those children each wanted to have the letter read to his or her own group. The letters describe the complexity of depression as it is experienced by the writer, as well as what it feels like to hold on to depressive affect.

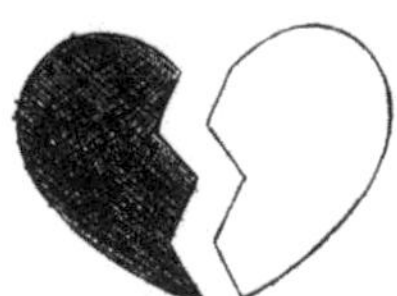

Letter #1

The first letter was submitted by Gillian in Girls' Group #3. She wrote it in an individual treatment session with Dr. DeGangi.

> *Dear Girls' Group,*
>
> I am feeling so sad and I do not know why. Someone can tell me something that is sad and I feel like crying. Other times, I feel really in the dumps, like my life isn't worth living. I even cry in my pillow at night sometimes, but I don't always have a reason for crying. I also have outbursts over little things. When I get angry, I have a major temper tantrum and I have troubles stopping. I feel moody a lot of the time. I also worry about things that don't seem important to anyone else. I don't really understand all this. I feel

like I am on a mood roller coaster. Does anybody else in your group feel like I do? What do you think this is about? Can anybody help me? Please.

Signed,
Peggy.

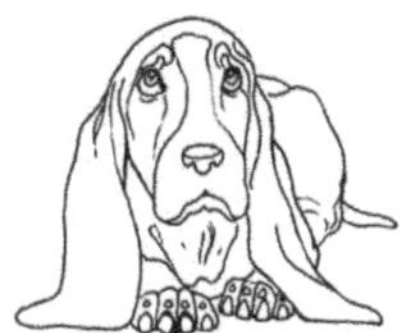

Letter #2

GD: Julian, a member of Boys' Group #2, wrote the following letter. His peers would pick on him mercilessly. They labeled him "gay" and when the letter was written, he was suffering a great deal from the depression he experienced after being ostracized by peers. He came for group one day with his letter folded tightly into a bundle. He handed it to me discreetly in the waiting room and whispered, "Please read this in group today."

Dear Boys' Club,

I have a problem with some kids I know. Don't even try telling me to fight them because they would beat the snot out of me. They call me gay and say I like girl things. This hurts me because I was trying to be friendly and I thought they were my friends. They really get under my skin and they know it and take advantage of it. I hate putting up with this stuff. Please give me some advice.

From,
Larry, the taunted

Boys' Group #2

Ian: Larry, I'm basically like you only I'm able to put up with a lot more stuff than you. Friends can be a bit of a pain sometimes, but not most of the time. Just ignore them. That's what I learned a long time ago.

Therapist: Even if they keep coming after you?

GD: I was pushing Ian a little in order to keep the issue alive.

MN: Ian was trying to come up with a quick solution for the letter-writer and stop the group process.

GD: I didn't want a showstopper.

Ian: Yeah, even if they keep coming after you. Just say, "Believe what you want to believe, but you don't know me."

Therapist: That's a really good suggestion.

Ian: Unless they do know you, then say, "Think what you want to think. I don't care." Let it go. Go with the flow.

Julian: Actually, I think that this guy has already tried ignoring from the sound of it.

GD: It's interesting that Julian said this, because it's clearly not in the letter. Since he was the letter-writer, what he said was a bit more publicly self-revealing. It showed that he was in-the-know.

MN: Within the group dynamic, he responded directly to Ian: "This letter-writer has tried your suggestion and it doesn't work."

Therapist: Then give some other advice.

Kevin: I get a lot of death threats from this kid and he keeps saying that he's going to kill me. He tries to choke me. I try to run away as fast as I can. He whacks me on the head with a book. He gets angry at me for no apparent reason and he says he's going to kill me. I just tell him that "This is getting really old and boring. OK. You're going to kill me. I've heard that before. Can you come up with something new before I lose interest completely?" I just act indifferent around him.

MN: That was a sophisticated response.

GD: Despite his Asperger's, Kevin had done very well as he had matured. He had some good internal resources to call on.

Aidan: You said to tell them that you're getting bored of what they're saying. If they keep on calling you one word, they can think of other words that are just as annoying to you. You'll be in school with them for a while. Put up with them while you can. When Julian said that maybe they already tried ignoring, keep on ignoring them until it works. It doesn't matter if you already tried it and you think it doesn't work. I have a little retarded asshole in my class who is pissing me off. I am trying to ignore him. He's just messed up. I say, "I'm higher than them." They try to threaten me and call me gay. They're using words like that. They probably feel bad that they're gay themselves.

Therapist: All the same, Aidan, it's tough to keep on having that said to you.

GD: I personalized my comment. I was trying to empathize with Aidan to convey the message that one doesn't have to put up with this and do it alone.

Therapist: You try ignoring and blocking it off, it still offends you. And Kevin, you said that they're physically bothering you.

GD: Youngsters like those in this group don't have the emotional stamina or social skills to fight back in healthy ways when other children, who have so much emotional and physical aggression, pick on them. It's hard to sustain a defense against that. I really feel for them.

MN: It's so hard at this age. These developmentally compromised children are really very vulnerable. More intact kids are better able to deflect what comes their way, although it's still not easy.

GD: All the children in this group were easy targets.

Kevin: He's been my ex-friend on and off. I don't know if he's a friend or an enemy. He's the most hated enemy of a friend. He keeps on trying to choke me and it's not like something you can ignore.

Julian: I was going to say that I convinced my friend to write this letter and I gave it to Georgia. I know what's going on with him. He says it's not going on in school.

GD: Julian was admitting to the group that he had given the letter to me, but he was saying it as many people do: "I have this friend who . . . ."

Ian: Kids can be mean to you sometimes. They can piss you off. Even if it's your friends, then just ignore them.

Therapist: If someone says something that hurts you a lot, like you're called "gay," how do you convince yourself inside that you're not, even though you're hearing it from other kids?

GD: I wanted to bring out what happens to a person internally when he keeps hearing something negative about himself from others.

MN: Again this is the therapeutic question: whether to pursue material or not. The therapist has to put this through the gristmill of her mind. Being called "gay" at this age is quite common and is intended to be very hurtful. I'm not sure, though, if when kids say it they mean it literally. It would be good for the therapist to clarify this point to the children because their social thinking is not very clear. The intent is mean-spirited, but the specific words may not actually matter. Nevertheless, they sting.

Kevin: I tell them that they're mentally retarded.

Aidan: Get someone to tell you that you're not.

GD: He resonated to my comment.

MN: The whole group was "resonant" right then.

Manuel: I just ignore them.

Therapist: How do you make it better inside when you hear this awful stuff? That's the part I'm concerned about it. If someone hurls an insult at me, I have to do something about the damage that it caused to me inside.

GD: This time I personalized my comment so that the internal experience of being damaged would stay alive in the room.

Kevin: Insult them.

GD: Kevin externalized and deflected it. My comment pushed him to a place that he couldn't tolerate.

Therapist: I wouldn't insult them back because that fuels the problem. I'm talking about what happens inside. You're still getting damaged.

Manuel: I just think of other stuff. Something fun.

GD: That fell flat and ended the group's discussion.

MN: It fell flat but I think Manuel was speaking for the group: "We're talking about these hurtful things and we can't do it any more. End of subject."

GD: Manuel was a walled-off child, who usually sat with a blank look on his face, and rarely responded. The fact that he said "I just think of other stuff" may have reflected what he did all the time. Throughout the group sessions, he rarely had a voice. We've rarely heard from him in these transcripts.

MN: In group therapy with children who are compromised, a therapist often needs to engage in a degree of self-disclosure that we would not ordinarily do. I think it needs to be done to join with them in order for them to feel not so alone. Therapist self-disclosure also grounds the youngsters in a realistic experience that we ourselves have had. By doing this, we are implicitly saying that they're not so different from us and we're not so different from them, in contextually relevant ways.

So we do share much, much more about ourselves than we might with other, less developmentally compromised, youngsters in a group.

GD: Exactly. In a group of kids who are so vulnerable, I like to use myself as a clarifying voice. I frequently will pull out something that I'm willing to say to help them along. I don't think I'm revealing a whole lot about myself, just enough to provide security and safety in talking more about the topic. I use self-disclosure to clarify what the real issue is and what are some responses that a person might have. It's a way to humanize the identification that we are all in this together. We all suffer from these things because we are human.

Letter #3

The letter that follows is about a child who feels overwhelmed with sadness when socially rejected. It was written to provide a forum for discussing depression. This letter was written by the anonymous therapist, not by any group member.

Dear Kids' Club,

I have a couple of things that I want to tell you. I have a really good friend, Brendan (Brenda in girl's version), who I like a lot. We have fun together and share a lot of interests in common. I can really talk to him when things are bothering me. He is my best friend. Recently Brendan has been playing with other kids on the playground and sometimes when I call him to get together, he says that he's busy with other friends. I can't tell you how rejected I feel! I don't like anyone else in the way I like him. It's really hard for me to make new friends and I feel completely betrayed by him. Doesn't he like me too? I thought we were best buddies all these years. I am feeling left out, rejected, and very sad. I don't feel like doing anything anymore. What do you think I should do about this?

Signed,
Ray, the Rejected
(Becky in girl's version)

MN: This sounds like a youngster who was not able yet to enter into a more enlarged social world as he approached adolescence. He interpreted the normal behavior of a friend who was enlarging his world as a complete rejection rather than adding himself to Brendan's new collection of friends. However, it is possible that Brendan was truly not responding to Ray. Hopefully the youngsters listening to this letter talked about that rejection.

GD: Many children coming in for therapy at 11, 12, and 13 years old experience this shift in their friendship groups. They don't know how to be resourceful enough to find new friends. Their social world is small. In normal development, children are building resilience and finding second and third "families" in various peer groups at this period.

Girls' Group #2

Chelsea: Almost the same thing happened to me. What I did was for a few weeks I completely pretended that that person was invisible and let them do what they want.

Then you go back and say, "You've been ignoring me." Sometimes if you really start talking with them and try to get together with them, just don't let it get to you and don't think that they don't like you anymore. They may have friends that they've had for a long time.

MN: Chelsea was doing well initially when she started to speak about the problem. She was using imaging as a technique, imagining that the offending person is invisible, that nobody was there. She felt the freedom not to be hurt because nobody was there to hurt her. However, she then fell back and lost her resourcefulness; she couldn't pull it off.

Annie: In preschool there was this person named Sarah. I wanted to play with her and I would follow her around and be annoying. Then I started ignoring her and finally she wanted to play with me.

MN: Perhaps Annie was turning the tables by rejecting the friend and she thought that it worked. There have now been two girls in a row who came up with strategies that they attempted. By middle school, though, these solutions wouldn't work any more.

GD: Annie had a tendency to be intrusive to others. She was able to break that pattern and learned to back away from the friend.

MN: There was also a backing-away that both Annie and Chelsea did by placing events in the past.

Therapist: It helps that you had the same problem and what you learned was that backing off a little might have helped.

Briana: What usually helps me is do what they want back. I'm best friends with someone and I hang out with them, but at lunch and recess I let her play with her other friends. I find other friends to play with too. I really like to play with the boys. I go see if there's anybody else to play with.

GD: Briana brought it to the present, which is what I hoped would happen, and in some ways she showed that she understood the problem in this letter. It was a healthy response that was unusual for her. When we've looked at other letter sessions, we've seen that Briana typically didn't contribute to the discussions.

MN: The issue of rejection brought her out.

Maya: You could go do what your friend is doing. Try it for a day or two and if you like it, keep doing that. You could also make a deal with your friend. At lunch she could play with whoever she wants half the time, then the other half the time play with you.

Ellen: I have a problem like this. All my friends want to spend time with me but some of them don't like each other. They're really annoying and get mad at me when I say, "I want to play with whomever." I just try to compromise.

Therapist: Compromise is a big part of this.

GD: I was surprised to hear Ellen describe herself as the center of attention when she was usually shy and withdrawn. Something did not ring true in her response. She seemed to be acting as if she were not the injured party when, in fact, she was just like the child in this letter.

MN: She saw herself as the child in the letter and had to quickly make herself not be that child. This was a flight into a state that she could tolerate. Rejection, in that moment, was intolerable to her.

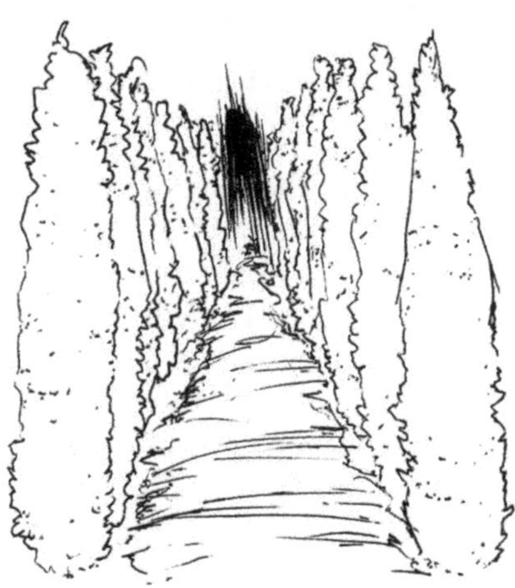

Girls' Group #3

Ashley: I think that you should go over and ask her what the matter is. Why she isn't friends with you anymore and ask if you did something to make her avoid you. Tell her you're sorry and can you please be friends again?

Therapist: You're right. She may have offended her friend in some way and doesn't know what she did.

Ashley: You probably didn't know that you offended her. Invite her over. When you're alone, she might be nicer. She might like to get to know other people, too.

Therapist: Maybe she's not just a one-friend person.

MN: Ashley was making a good point: you might have pushed your friend away. On the other hand, she was not able to tolerate that the rejection had occurred at all because she suggested inviting the girl over. The sequence betrayed her.

GD: Ashley had merged two discrepant concepts—avoidance of rejection with approach: "Be my friend." Ashley was a socially adept child so her thought process surprised me.

MN: I think we have seen a minor failure of ego-integration. The rejection aspect of the letter troubled Ashley, so she fragmented her thinking and became less able to conceptualize this in a logical way.

GD: When a child like Ashley says something like this, it appears that her emotional flooding derails her cognitive capacities.

MN: This can happen to most people in the right, or should I say wrong, circumstances.

Deborah: Her friend may be wanting to fit in. Maybe she's not very popular and she is ashamed and wants to fit in. She doesn't want to be weird with only one friend.

Ashley: She may also be grumpy now.

MN: Deborah and Ashley demonstrated a potential for empathy in this conversation. They also demonstrated that capacity by putting themselves in the rejecting friend's shoes and trying to understand what reason there might be for the rejecting behavior. While they wouldn't solve the problem, their responses showed the capacity for these youngsters to respond empathically in the group, a capacity that could go beyond the scope of the letters.

GD: What I also like is that Ashley was bringing up that the girl can feel grumpy and that this could set her off even more, resulting in more social distancing.

Therapist: Have any of you been on the other side of the coin where you have a tag-along friend who becomes a pest to you?

Ashley: Yeah, one of my friends is nice, then other times is very annoying. She doesn't like everything I like to do. When I'm with her I have to do whatever she wants to do. She was also very annoying and jumped all over me. "What do you want to do now? Can I show you something?" I'd say, "Hold on. Let me finish this." She really bugged me. I'm not mean to her, but I just pretend that I'm annoyed.

Alexis: I have a little monkey that's always attached to me at school. Her name is Rose and she runs up and hugs me so hard that she almost broke my ribs. She's a second grader.

GD: In reflecting on this conversation and looking at my response as the therapist, I'm uncertain why I chose to bring out the opposite problem—that is, when someone has a pesky friend who bothers her. I must have been responding to something in the room.

MN: I'd like to make a guess. You might have been responding to a non-verbal cue or an unarticulated feeling. I think that Ashley and Alexis were putting themselves in the rejected person's shoes and you went right into "Has this ever happened to you?" I think this raises a point that we don't always like to admit. As therapists we aren't always conscious of why we're saying what we're saying. We usually like to be very careful about what we're saying, but sometimes we can't articulate a reason for it.

GD: As you and I have read these transcripts together, I often remembered something that was happening in the group room at the time. Something that was unspoken, like the child who scratched on the table nervously while we were talking, or the child who laughed uncontrollably as a defensive response. Those were dramatic examples of non-verbal and affective responses that steer the therapist's ship. This time I don't remember anything specific, but I must have been tuning into something non-verbal.

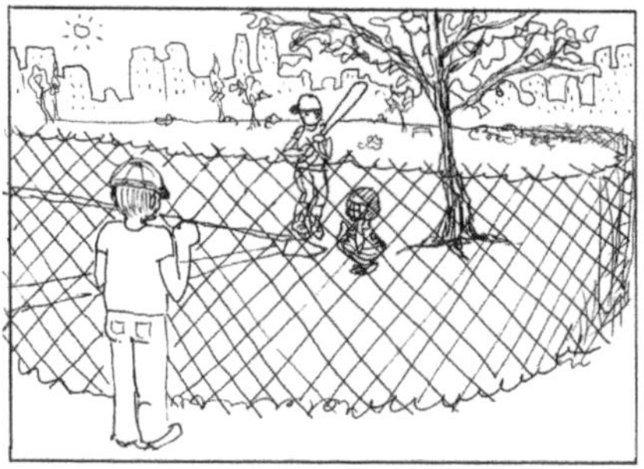

Girls' Group #4

Caitlin: As you said in your letter, I feel that same way too. I also feel when I'm around Vanessa and she doesn't want to be my friend anymore. I think she doesn't want to be my friend ever again. It rips my heart out.

Therapist: Does she know it rips your heart out?

Caitlin: Yes.

Therapist: And she still rejects you?

Caitlin: Yes. And she plays with her other friends. I still like her so much. She's the only person that I love at school.

MN: This hit her hard!

GD: Yes, it did.

MN: She was first identifying, and then she went into elaborating very painfully what it felt like to be her. It seems that she got stuck. She fell into the abyss and her heart was "ripped" because of the rejection. I'd like to see if she had the resources to find a solution, either internal so that her heart wouldn't feel ripped, or an external social solution that put her in a better position as she related to others.

GD: I was aware of how emotionally overwrought she was, and I wanted to see if she could plan a cognitive strategy.

Therapist: Have you found anything to help with this problem when she's playing with other kids?

Caitlin: Find someone else. Try to get along with them. "Hello, my name is Becky, and what's your name?" You might get along with them. So that's my advice.

GD: Isn't it lovely; she was giving advice to herself.

Therapist: Advice for Becky and advice for you. Any other ideas for when you're left out? (No response) Does it help you, Caitlin, to know that other kids in this world feel the same way that you do?

Caitlin: (Giggles)

MN: What kind of giggling was that?

GD: It was a falling-apart, disjointed, and disorganized giggling.

MN: So it was actually an ego-failure during which she wasn't able to speak in words. Caitlin had been fairly articulate until then, but became overwhelmed and unable to speak.

GD: I'd like to say something about the group process. This letter had an open impact on only one child in the group, but if we look at Caitlin's responses over time, she was participating and learning about herself and others through these letters. She was maturing and developing some insights and resources.

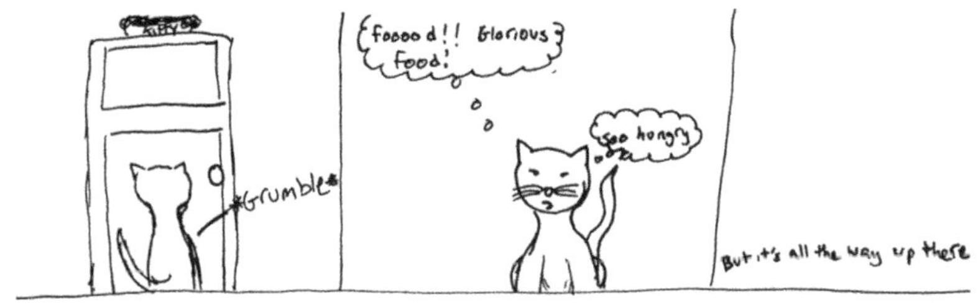
Grumble
Foooo d!! Glorious Food!
Soo hungry
But it's all the way up there

Activities

1. Write down on a piece of paper without anyone seeing, the "most embarrassing thing that ever happened to you." Fold it and give it to the group leader to read anonymously and open up discussion. Other follow-up activities may be to write down "The best day of my life was . . ." or "The worst day of my life was . . . ."
2. Play a game where each child starts putting five fingers in the air. Going around the room, each child says something that they have never done and that they think nobody has done. For example, if a child says, "I have never dived off a diving board" and four others have, they put down a finger. The child with the most fingers up in the air at the end of the game wins.
3. Tell about a time when you felt sad. What set off feeling sad?
   a. Things turning out badly
   b. Not getting what you wanted
   c. Losing a friendship
   d. Missing somebody
   e. Being rejected or excluded
   f. Being disliked by others
   g. Being with someone who is sad, hurt, or in pain.
4. When you are sad, what does it feel like in your body?
   a. Feel tired and run down
   b. Want to stay in bed all day
   c. Feel there's nothing fun or pleasurable any more
   d. Feel empty
   e. Cry
   f. Don't want to eat
   g. Troubles sleeping
   h. Get grouchy.

Have children show what they look like when they are sad and how they sound when they talk. Then follow-up with "what helps when you feel sad?"

References

DeGangi, G. A. (2000). *Pediatric disorders of regulation in affect and behavior: A therapist's guide to assessment and treatment*. New York: Academic Press.

Geller, B. & DelBello, M. P. (2003). *Bipolar disorder in childhood and early adolescence*. New York: Guilford Press.

Greenspan, S. I. (2003). *The secure child: Helping our children feel safe and confident in a changing world*. Cambridge, MA: DeCapo.

Greenspan, S. I. & Glovinsky, I. (2002). *Bipolar patterns in children: New perspectives on developmental pathways and a comprehensive approach to prevention and treatment*. Bethesda, MD: Interdisciplinary Council for Developmental and Learning Disorders.

CHAPTER 20

Look Out! I'm Going to Explode!

Children with mood dysregulation usually have significant problems with anger control. These youngsters suffer from a chronic state of irritability that is easily exacerbated by over-stimulation, transitions in activities, and task and situational demands. A dysregulated child's difficulty resolving social conflicts can cause increased agitation. Once the anger reaches a certain threshold, he explodes into a tantrum, and may be inconsolable for a long period of time. He is unable to calm himself or to use strategies that could lead to a decrease in the discharge of anger. Often the mood-dysregulated child cannot predict which situations will serve as a trigger, and simultaneously cannot accurately read those body cues that signal the onset of anger in self and others (Greene, 2001; Miklowitz & Goldstein, 1997; Turecki, 2000). The letter in this chapter attempts to capture the unregulated child's complex experience of anger.

Dear Kids' Club,

I have a really huge anger problem. All kinds of things bug me. Before I know it, kaboom! I have launched into a really big rage, throwing things, kicking anyone near me, and yelling foul things to my parents, kids at school, or anyone in earshot. I'll give you a few examples of what sets me off. I can be at school getting irritated by this kid who sits next to me. Fred does this thing when he multi-tasks—doing more than one thing at a time and doing it in fast motion. Like he's packing up his bag, snacking on his fruit roll-up that he hides in his desk, talking to me, raising his hand to the teacher to ask a question, then he's back making his homework list. It drives me crazy! After watching that for a few days, I broke into a real rage! They had to clear the classroom of everyone because I threw desks over, smashed a few things, and yelled like it was nobody's business.

Here's another example of what could set me off. I can be playing a board game with my little brother at home. As usual, he's winning, the little brat! It's a total humiliation when I'm four years older than him. He's a big bragger when he wins, doing his stupid touchdown dance. He was beating me at checkers and I blew up. I threw the pieces around the room, screamed at him, and hit him on the head with the board. It's only cardboard so it couldn't have hurt him bad, but he was screaming like I had used a cinder block. What a little creep! Of course, I'm the one who gets in big trouble.

My mom threw me in my bedroom, then when I called her a "bitch," she said, "That's it, bucko! You just lost TV for the month!"

Anyway, I do these blow-ups almost every day, sometimes several times a day. Does anyone in your group know about what this is like? What have you done that works?

Signed,
Andrew, the Angry One
(Angie in girl's version)

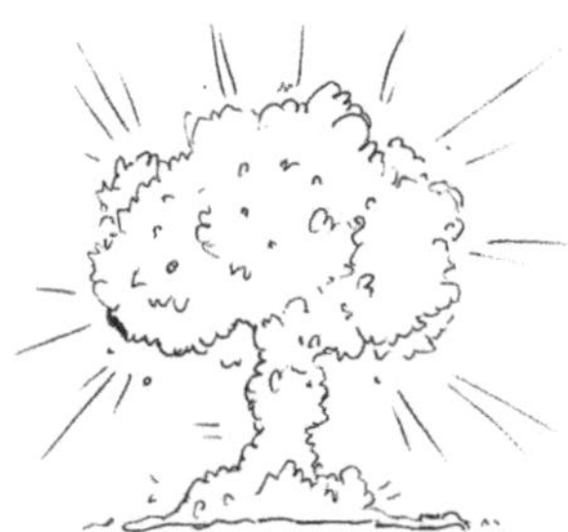

Boys' Group #1

Duncan: This Andrew person is a crazy person and he'll end up getting arrested one day. It's a real horror story. He's like these kids you read about in the news who have a horrible attitude and finally he has had it and then kills them all.

MN: He was quite frightened by the level of aggression in the letter.

Therapist: You're thinking about what happened in the news this week? The boy who was so rageful that he did some harmful things to people.

GD: I brought up what had happened in the news that week because any current event like that does pollute the group; it brings something in from the "outside." A boy had gone into a mall and used a gun to shoot into the crowd. It made the news quite dramatically.

Manuel: One thing is that you need to take a "chill" pill. It means "relax." Just because someone is multi-tasking doesn't mean they're a bad person. I multi-task. I can easily walk, drink a soda, and chew gum at the same time. Life sucks when your little sibling does the victory dance. It will get better when he finally gets to be mature. To tell you the truth, you need to be more mature as well and you need to stop throwing temper tantrums just because things aren't going your way.

Therapist: Let's not assume that he's immature. Let's assume that these are the things that really get to him. What can he do to calm down? And he does want to know if any of you in here have a short fuse.

GD: I thought that chalking the letter-writer's behavior up to immaturity would be unhelpful to the group. It could have gotten them off-the-hook in terms of talking about the real issues. I also wanted to depart from the idea of "just knock it off! Just snap out of it!" This is something a lot of parents do with their children when they fall apart. Manuel sounded very parental to me.

MN: Parentified and lacking empathy. The youngster in this letter knows that his behavior is not acceptable; that's why he's writing his letter. Manuel's solution would cause the young letter-writer to lose face and feel lectured at and not listened to. Nothing would be gained. You were aware of that, so you pulled the group back to problem-solving and thinking about itself.

Javier: I only have one thing to say. Go to a psychologist!
Therapist: That's actually good advice.
Manuel: (Laughing) He's a nut case!
Therapist: How would a psychologist help him?

GD: I wanted to put them in the psychologist's shoes.
MN: I sometimes literally change places with a youngster, which is what you're thinking about here. I'm taking your thought a little bit farther. For instance, something might be present in the child's play material and I would say: "You know what? Let's trade places right now. I'm going to be Johnny and you're going to be Dr. Nemiroff. Let's do what we just did again and this time you try to help me." The kids enjoy it and try to find ways to be helpful to themselves when it's acted out in this way. Interestingly, the kids usually know exactly what you're up to, and they love it.
GD: That technique is very effective and can be transformational to some children. They suddenly see the other side.
MN: In doing a technique like that, the therapist has to be like the youngster, but never completely imitative, nor crossover into anything that might feel to the child that you're making fun of him.

Javier: He would help you control your anger. (Manuel is still laughing)
Therapist: Maybe your advice is to go to someone who will help you find some strategies that will work.
Jacob: About the little brother who does the victory dance. Somehow make it be that you win sometimes and you do the victory dance.

MN: That response exposed Jacob's level of immaturity.

Therapist: Are you suggesting that in order to get revenge on the little brother? (Jacob said "yes"). The other reason to do a victory dance is because you might want the brother to know how you feel. That's a very different reason to do it.

GD: I wanted to see if I could pull Jacob into a more mature response.

Jacob: You should do it so that you want the little brother to know how it feels.
Duncan: He's way more than psycho. He's a criminal. I have a feeling that he's already a murderer.

GD: Duncan was still distraught about the events of the week. He was sitting in the corner and folding his ears in on themselves. He literally took the outside of his ear and folded it into the inside of the ear canal. He desperately needed to shut out what he was hearing.
MN: It was an auditory flight response.

Tyrone: Sometimes even if your brother beats you in a game, it's not the end of the world. Watch what he does and try to beat him in the same strategy he uses.

GD: The group got stuck on getting revenge; I wanted to re-direct them.

Therapist: How many boys in here have blown their top? All of you except Duncan.

Duncan: I have a really good sense of humor and I use that to help me.

GD: Duncan had Asperger's syndrome and he would sometimes show a quirky sense of humor. But I also don't think he understood or completely followed all of the conversation here.

Therapist: That's a good strategy, instead of snapping at the person. Can I hear one or two suggestions for him?

Manuel: Like I said earlier, mostly find a game that you're good at and that your brother isn't good at. Tell him, "Now your life sucks. I'm the best. Go run to mom and see what she says about me winning. Ha!" Also see a criminal psychologist.

Tyrone: Sometimes if you go and tell your mom, think about that he's younger than you and you have learned that it's not right to be a poor sport.

MN: That was a nice way for Tyrone to end the group because he was getting away from seeing a criminal psychologist. The group was thinking of what had happened that week—the shooting at that mall. A space that should have felt safe, a mall, was penetrated by danger in an uncontrolled way. That was very frightening. Tyrone ended the group by seeking out someone, his mom, who was safe. He got quite logical. This was useful to the group.

GD: I like ending groups that have been emotionally distraught with something organizing. It grounds the group and they leave more put-together both on an emotional and physiological level. Especially when groups have had shared a traumatic experience, I don't want them leaving in an emotionally activated state.

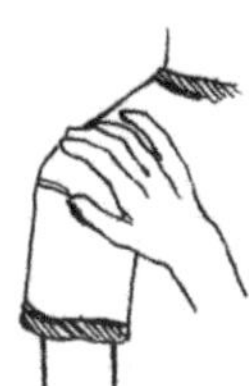

Letter #2

The next letter was written by Greer, a member of Girls' Group #5. She wrote the letter confidentially and asked the group leader to read it to the group. She gave the letter-writer an anonymous name and did not disclose her identity.

GD: Greer was the child whose mother was blind and whose father had a coping deficit. Father looked like a street person and his wife could not see it. Greer was quite upset that no one knew what her life was like because nobody else had a blind mother. She had recently been diagnosed with bipolar disorder. Her uncle also was bipolar and had had constant strife in his life, so Greer worried about what it meant to be bipolar. I'm struck by the fact that she didn't speak in the discussion that follows. I think that she was just taking it in.

Dear Girls' Group,

I am always so mean to every one in my family. This is especially my little brothers. I want to stop, but I don't know if I can. I need help really badly.

Your friend,
Lily

Girls' Group #5

Therapist: Do any of you ever find yourself being mean and you don't know why?

Nadia: Once I was really mean to my parents. I don't know why. Then I said, "Why am I so angry?" I thought about it and realized it was that I had had a really bad day and I was taking it out on my mom and dad.

MN: This is very mature. Nadia was demonstrating the ability to observe herself. This was a lovely way to start the group. In the moment, I'd be watching to see if the group used her observing ego as the model for that session.

GD: It was uncharacteristic of Nadia to say something so insightful.

Therapist: So you thought that what was happening was that it wasn't really about your parents, but that there was something that was difficult for you like you had a long day.

Jacqueline: Sometimes this kid in my class does things like pushes over my papers. I yelled at him, "Jacob, why did you do that?" and he said, "I didn't mean to." I just yelled at him before I had time to think. I'm probably going to say something to him tomorrow about it.

Therapist: It just flew out of your mouth before you realized.

MN: The group was continuing to be able to use an observing ego. Jacqueline was reflecting upon what she did. Nadia's opening response was helpful to Jacqueline.

GD: Jacqueline was the type of child who needed to think things over before she responded. She needed lead time to think about what she would do the next day.

Brooke: I tell my classmates, if they're really having a problem, "Just stop! Try not to do it. It may be a reaction, but break the reaction. You have to take hold of yourself, and tell yourself to stop it. They're people you love, right? If you love them, then try to stop yelling at them. Try to put you in their shoes and think how they feel when you yell at them. Try to get some courage and say you're sorry. It really hurts their feelings."

GD: I experienced a strong counter-transference reaction to Brooke. When she would talk like this, I wanted to stop listening and flee. Brooke was so narcissistic and would often pontificate on what others should or shouldn't do.

MN: I had the same reaction. The content sounded adaptive, but there was something about it that nevertheless sounded empty.

GD: The empty part was "Just snap out of it! Just stop!" There was no emotional connection between the action and the interaction with others. It was almost like she was outside the main process of the group.

MN: It sounded empathic, but it really wasn't.

GD: It was sermonizing. The girls responded by distancing themselves from her. None of them liked her.

Nadia: Sometimes when I'm really mad at my parents for no reason, it is sometimes because I have too much homework. I can't get it all done and not enough time to do it. Then I get mad at my parents.

Brooke: Don't take it out on other people. Let's just say that Brittany yelled at me because I colored her face half pink and half green or with lipstick and stuff. Then she yells at me. Then I take my anger out on my parents. Then I'd be wasting my energy in the wrong place.

Brittany: You can also get yourself a little punching bag and take it out on that. Also, my mom gets mad at my dog, Figgy, my dad, and at me. You can get mad at your loved ones, but they should know you still love them. At least try punching a balloon that's filled with helium, not filled with air. Get a balloon that won't pop so easily. I used to break a #2 pencil. I wasn't a happy camper then. Now I am better with my anger.

MN: She was demonstrating her good use of displacement.

GD: Yes. And she was also talking about two specific things. Her mother would lose control and Brittany's job was to contain it. It was very hard for her. Secondly, she was a child who had been abused, traumatized, and abandoned by her biological and foster parents. She had a huge amount of anger that she had to contain. Displacement was one way.

MN: She was telling the truth here? "I wasn't a happy camper then, and now I'm better with my anger."

GD: Yes. She was in a better home situation, even though she now had a mother who would discharge anger. Brittany was overwhelmed by it and didn't know what to do with it.

MN: Are you talking about this in the Winnicott sense of containing? She had to be the parent to the youngster's (but in this case, her mother's) feelings? She had to hold inside herself the feelings her mother couldn't tolerate? (GD: "Yes.")

GD: This letter brought up the kinds of angry feelings that are unique to a child with a bipolar disorder. It is a progressive illness that begins to show itself in childhood, usually middle adolescence, and then worsens and gets more extreme at both ends of the mood spectrum—the manic and depressive aspects of the illness. Medication needs to be monitored and usually increased. Greer was 12 at the time, a typical time for bipolar illness to be diagnosed.

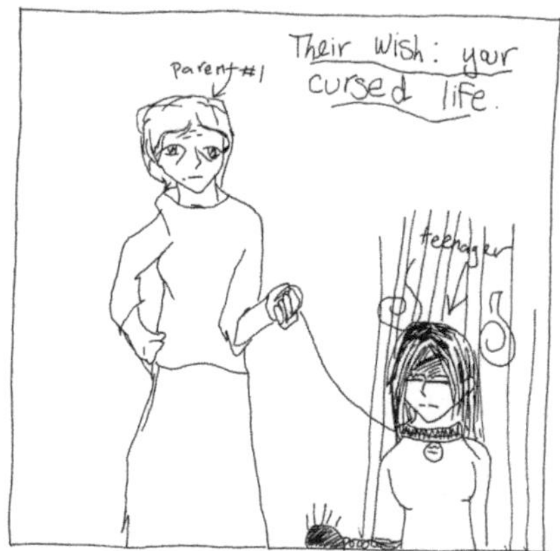

Activities

1. Construct an add-on story using small miniatures or other props about feeling angry. Children can either act-out the story, tell it, or enact it using a sand table.

2. Make a board game using markers and a large poster board. Each child comes up with a land of their own. When other children land their mover on their "land," the child draws cards that tell them to do things or answer questions. Have file cards available for youngsters to write down "challenges" for the interlopers, such as "Write your name with your toes on a piece of paper" or to answer questions like "If you were on a desert island, which three people or things would you want with you?"
3. Have each child describe what happens when they express their anger. Here is a list of some possibilities:
   a. Get out of control
   b. Feel tight in body
   c. Feel like going to explode
   d. Teeth clamp together
   e. Cry, unable to stop tears
   f. Want to hit, bang the wall, throw something, blow up
   g. Face gets red
   h. Curse and use obscenities
   i. Use a loud voice, yell or shout
   j. Pound on something, throw things, break things
   k. Stomp, slam doors.

Follow-up by talking about how they feel after they have been angry. For instance, do they think about it over and over again and cannot get it out of their mind? Do they think about how they will get revenge? Do they have constructive strategies, such as figuring out how to negotiate the problem with the other persons? Then move into how the child self-calms and constructive ways to express anger (i.e., punch a pillow, play the drums, and exercise).

References

Greene, R. W. (2001). *The explosive child: A new approach for understanding and parenting easily frustrated, chronically inflexible children* (2nd ed.). New York: HarperCollins.

Miklowitz, D. J. & Goldstein, M. J. (1997). *Bipolar disorder: A family-focused treatment approach*. New York: Guilford Press.

Turecki, S. (with Tonner, L.). (2000). *The difficult child* (2nd ed.). New York: Bantam Books.

CHAPTER 21
Wringing My Hands!

Children who are consumed with anxiety spend their time feeling upset and overwhelmed over everyday tasks that are usually effortless for other children. Anxieties take many forms. Fears about everyday experiences or events such as bugs, dogs, thunderstorms, or a circus clown may distress a child. Some children worry about performing tasks, obsessing about how they have done, to the point that quick tasks end up taking a very long time. Some children have performance anxiety and panic during test-taking or when speaking or performing in front of a group. Then there are children who anxiously do not want to leave their parents to go to school or visit a friend; such youngsters might refuse to speak or develop a phobia about going to school. Often these anxieties affect a youngster's ability to concentrate on tasks and to tolerate being alone. Sleep disturbances often develop as worries become magnified by the darkening night. Nightmares or recurring "bad dreams" about fears can dominate and disrupt sleep.

The causes of anxiety in children range from constitutional "hard-wiring" that predisposes the nervous system to intensified anxiety, to potentially traumatizing events, or environmental stressors. Regardless of the cause, the child feels insecure and unsafe. Physical aches and pains such as stomachaches or headaches may develop as the child seeks to avoid situations that cause agitation. Panic attacks may also develop when external conditions are such that the child cannot cope (Annunziata & Nemiroff, 2009; Brooks & Siegel, 1996; DeGangi & Kendall, 2008; Rapoport, 1989).

This chapter focuses on two types of anxiety. The first letter addresses performance anxiety. The second letter describes a child who worries at night and cannot sleep because he feels unsafe or thinks something bad will happen to him.

Letter #1: Performance Anxiety

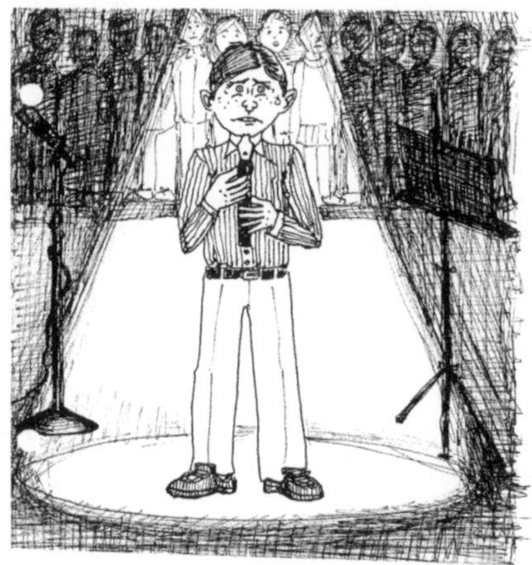

Dear Kids' Club,

I don't know about you guys, but I get really wrecked out about tests. I usually don't study until the day before, and then I cram information into my head. I remember well, so when I go into the exam, the information is all there. Here's what happens. I sit down and look at the test paper and my heart starts pounding, my palms are sweating, and my head feels like it's going to explode. Sometimes it gets so bad I can barely breathe. I look out the window and get this weird sensation like this isn't real. Sometimes I do OK on the test, but other times I don't and my mom and dad say, "What happened, you knew that?" The other problem that goes with this is I freak out when I have to talk in front of the class, like read a paper that I wrote. The same thing happens to my body. I chew on my fingernails and pick at my skin a lot just thinking about these things. If I could get out of tests and oral presentations for now on, I'd be fine, but I can't. I'm starting to hate school for this reason. I feel like a nervous wreck. What should I do?

Signed,
Norvin, the Nervous
(Nora in girl's version)

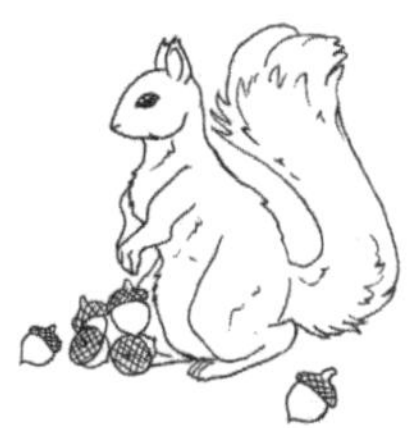

Girl's Group #3

Ashley: I get nervous when the teacher says there's a test next week. I say, "A test!! I don't like this!" Everybody always jokes and says, "She's going to freak out. You shouldn't have told her that." I guess I get more nervous than everybody else. Today I handed in an essay but I didn't realize that I had to staple the checklist on the back, so now my grade is only an A–. I was really nervous about it. Then the teacher said, "I'm reading a few examples of good ones" and then she read mine.

Deborah: Know what you have. It's called test anxiety and a lot of kids have it. It doesn't really have to do with whether you studied or not. It's just that when you see a test, you get really anxious and you think you're going to fail. Then you can't think of the answers anymore. Sometimes schools help kids with that by asking them the questions verbally or giving them a worksheet. The morning before the test they try to make the classroom a place that won't get them anxious like they turn on music. Maybe ask the teacher to do this or to give you the test in another form because it's just being anxious about the test and nothing else.

GD: It was a very practical solution: Here's your problem and this is what you do for it!

MN: It was also thought-out very logically before Deborah actually articulated it. She had really thought about this and tried to find her own way to function in a situation that was very hard for her. I would be interested in knowing if this capacity for effective problem-solving was seen in other areas of her life.

GD: It was quite unusual for Deborah to be this analytical about other persons' lives.

Alexis: I'm like the same way as you. How I calm down is I take a few deep breaths. The teacher also hands out gum that helps me calm down. We also listen to music, but the bad thing about the music is when everyone takes votes and it's the majority rules. The music could lose and it won't be played. We also have special teachers at my school and they give me more time and you can stop whenever you want.

GD: They were speaking about accommodations, but not what it was like to have performance anxiety. That overwhelmed them. As the therapist, I remember thinking that I should follow their process and not interfere because the kids were grabbing the microphone in an animated way.

MN: There's a difference between what Deborah was saying, which was about an accommodation that she could do for herself, and Alexis who was other-focused and using an external locus of control. Alexis was relying on the environment to support her rather than taking responsibility for herself, what she could personally do to take control of the problem. The group was still avoiding the panic.

Gillian: What my teacher does is because I have accommodations, she writes for me. If you start getting nervous, say, "I can do it. Only try your best." If you know it, just try your best. That's what my dad always says.

Elizabeth: If the teacher won't let you listen to music, then try to bring a CD player in and make sure that the music isn't rock 'n roll. The kids will know the songs and start singing in the middle of the class.

MN: The girls were taking turns showing their coping strategies. Deborah was the most sophisticated in organizing an internal locus of control. The group members really were not relating to each other. They were just taking turns.

GD: It was likely that this letter hit a little too close to home in its tone. It was close enough that it stopped these youngsters from functioning as a group. Interestingly, the following year this group process evolved into the girls wanting to practice upcoming performances in front of one another. These included solo singing for a talent show, performing an Irish jig, and reciting a Hebrew prayer in front of the congregation. The girls also wanted to play "beauty parlor," fixing one another's hairstyles and testing out makeup, all in the spirit of giving one another positive feedback about how they presented themselves to others.

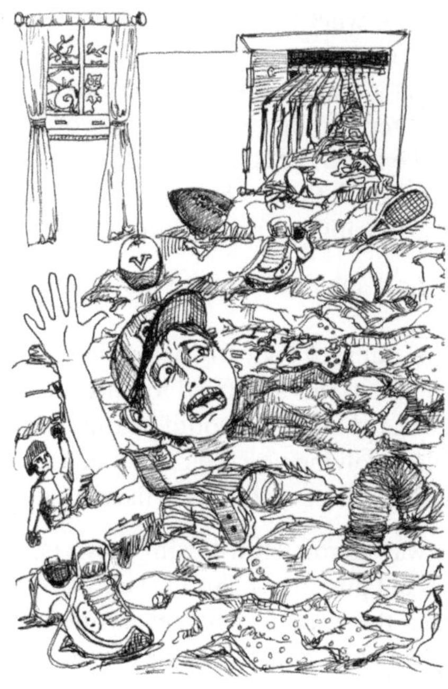

Boys' Group #3

Jamie: You could practice presenting in front of your parents. That would make it easier.

Therapist: What about the panic that he (the letter-writer) feels when he's standing in front of the class, the sweaty palms? Have any of you ever had this happened to you? Do any of you ever get nervous speaking in front of a group?

Jamie: I have stage fright. I do nothing. I just do it.

GD: I think he was saying that he forced himself through it.

MN: This was like the youngster in the previous group who said, "This is something I have to do and, therefore, rather than fight it, I'm going to forge ahead rather than struggle backwards."

Corey: I just pretend that the audience is just a bunch of ants. That helps me to pretend that.

GD: Corey was a boy who was paralyzed by anxiety. He had severe social anxiety and rarely spoke in his group.

MN: I think that he was getting close to addressing the panic in the letter. His strategy, which was a good one, was to reduce the audience, through imagery, to the size of a bunch of ants. Then he would not be talking to people anymore. He knew he was just pretending and it gave him the strength to carry on. He was the big person and he was just talking to little bugs. It gave him enough distance to be able to proceed.

GD: It was a very nice solution. I liked his use of visualization.

Oliver: Study early. This may sound ridiculous, but imagine all the people in their underwear. Then pray for our souls.

GD: This nicely humorous end of the group came from a boy who typically had been quite negative about himself. He was putting the audience in their underwear and that helped him gain distance. It permitted him to then do the task.

MN: This was a very nice process. I think that your one comment brings up three things that arise in the feeling-tone that accompanies anxiety. You used the words "panic, sweaty palms, and nervous." You did that in a way that was not heavy-handed, and so it helped the group to share some of the feelings about their own panic. This group's members, although they weren't talking directly to each other, were listening to each other and using each other's responses. These boys were resonating to each other in a very productive way.

Letter #2: Worries at Night

Dear Kids' Club,

I feel exhausted all the time because I can't sleep at night. Falling asleep is a big chore. I lay there thinking about how a person falls asleep and I pay attention to that moment when you actually shut down and it doesn't happen. I can lie there for hours before I finally fall asleep. My head starts to spin with worries about all kinds of things. I think that my dad might die because he looks old to me. I worry about how unsafe things are in the world. I get worked up about a terrorist attack (9/11) happening again and what will happen to me. Will I be with my mom and dad or will I be at school in a lock-down? I got started with these worries when the snipers were shooting people at gas stations and that kid at school. I laid down in the back seat of the car for weeks worried that he would get me too. I screamed at my mom to duck when she gassed up the car. I worry about all kinds of things. Sometimes I watch a scary movie and will think that someone is following me in my house or when I walk the dog.

No one knows how scared I feel inside. I'm afraid to tell anyone about it because boys aren't supposed to be afraid. My mom and dad think I'm just fine now that the sniper problem is over, but they have no idea. Sometimes they notice the dark circles under my eyes and say that I need to go to bed earlier, that I'm a kid who must need a lot of sleep. If they peek in my bedroom at night I pretend I'm sleeping. Does anyone in your group know about what a person does when they worry so much and are scared of bad things happening to them? I feel all jittery inside and don't know what to do.

Signed,
William, the Worrier
(Gwen in Girl's version)

Girls' Group #2

Briana: Sometimes I'm a big worrier. I worry when I'm near something that could happen. I used to worry about fires and people dying and things like that. Now, I've trained myself to focus on just what happens to me. I also sing to myself.

Sometimes when I'm scared, I torment my pillow. I used to torment my brother, but now I don't because he's nice now and it'll make him mean again if I torment him.

GD: Briana immediately talked about her worries in an open way. It was lovely.

MN: She could touch the feelings in this particular letter. Terrifying events had occurred in the Washington, D.C. area: the 9/11 terrorist attacks including sending a plane into the Pentagon; there was indeed a sniper shooting people at random and causing school lock-downs. These youngsters were better able to attach themselves to the feelings in the letter because of this. These were built-in shared experiences, realistically frightening events that these girls had to contend with in their daily lives. Briana, who in the past had avoided talking about feelings, could go right to it. She also brought up strategies that she had used and she was talking about some growth that she had had in the way she dealt with it. If I understood her correctly, there was a hint of humor in the use of the word "torment" twice. "I torment my pillow and I used to torment my brother." With that sense of humor, she was gaining some appropriate distance from her worry.

GD: This showed how therapists have to watch the use of individual words so carefully. At the time this letter was brought to the group, it was about one year after these youngsters were exposed to the random sniper who terrorized the Washington, D.C. area. I wondered about secondary trauma that they had probably experienced. They all knew trauma and were subjected to lock-downs in their schools when the sniper attacked the child on the school playground.

MN: Another interesting layer to this session was that the therapist experienced the same trauma. We were all present when the plane went into the Pentagon. We were all frightened of the sniper because he was operating right near where we live and work. It was happening right in front of us, very close to our homes and offices; even going to a gas station was frightening because the snipers were shooting people at random. This was a rather unusual situation: shared therapist/patient trauma, and therefore all the more important that the therapist be completely aware of his or her own responses to those traumatic incidences so that they don't leak into the group process.

Ellen: Sometimes I can't sleep at all. I count to ten over and over again. It puts me to sleep.

Chelsea: I have my very own stuffed animal collection and before I go to bed, I choose like five of my favorite stuffed animals. I choose my giant teddy bear and hug him very tight. He makes me feel very protected. If you're hugging something that makes you feel safe and warm.

GD: I was struck by her hugging a thing, not a person: that spoke to her difficulty attaching to people.

MN: It was another example of how you have to pay such close attention to the words that children use. She was coming up with a strategy, albeit immature, to hug a stuffed animal. She even used very young language—"my very own collection." Already that alerts us to the fact that she was emotionally functioning at a younger level. Then she talked about hugging a thing, as opposed to seeking the safety of nurturance from a person, ideally from a parent.

Therapist: Do any of you want to share what kinds of worries you have?

GD: Since the girls were so open already, I went a step further.

Ellen: I worry about murderers being in my closet.

Latisha: When I was younger, I was afraid that someone would come in my window or someone might come up behind me. Then I slept on my back.

Therapist: Do these worries ever creep back in? In the letter, the girl didn't tell her mom or dad about these worries. Do you think it would help her if she were to tell her parents that she has these fears?

GD: I wanted to bring in the aloneness of the worries.

MN: You also did something else that I think was unconsciously intuitive. You used the phrase "creep back in." This highlighted the sense of something happening insidiously, that it wouldn't be a robber bursting in the window but, rather, worries gradually slinking back in.

GD: That's the nature of anxiety—it is insidious and it is worse at night when people lie in beds and their brains ramble in the dark.

Briana: No. She might get in trouble. Whenever my friend's sister tells her parents and wants to sleep in her parents' bed, she gets spanked. Also, I used to be afraid of the window because there was a big tree outside. We were afraid that there was a guy out in the tree and he would shoot at us and kill us. We kept telling scary stories about the movie, then none of us could fall asleep.

GD: I think that by age 10, sleeping in the parents' bed for comfort and safety is not appropriate. That's what Briana was speaking about—getting spanked for sleeping with her parents in their bed.

MN: She was also describing the use of a counter-phobic defense. They were frightened of the guy out in the tree who would shoot and kill them. Then they told scary stories. Instead of trying to cope with their fear in a more rational manner, they moved toward the scary content. It kept them scared. It's the irony of the counter-phobic defense: it never works.

Ellen: If you can't sleep and you hear scary stuff, tell other people to tell something that's not scary.

GD: Here we have an isolated strategy, out of the blue. Ellen departed from the theme of worries. It was possible that the group discussion was more than she could tolerate.

Therapist: Something that helps when you have these kinds of scary thoughts is to focus on a safe and peaceful place. I still do that whenever something scary creeps into my head.

Emma: I think you really should tell someone. Sometimes when I get worried, I tell my parents, then I feel better.

Latisha: I think you should tell someone. You could get help and get suggestions for feeling better.

GD: This was interesting because in Latisha's individual therapy, she had a hard time articulating her fears. She could play about them through stories in the sand tray or use stuffed lizards and frogs to play out lock-down at school. She needed to play out her fears but could not articulate them as her own. It was OK for frogs to have scary feelings, but not Latisha herself.

MN: The group was functioning well. There was give-and-take, and, gradually, an ability to stay with the subject.

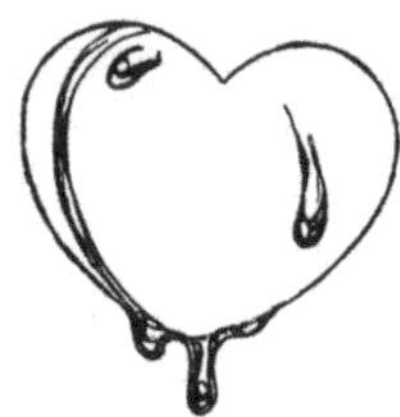

Boy's Group #3

Jamie: Don't watch so many monster movies at night. Read comic books instead. Also, we have a big army protecting us.

MN: Jamie's comment was a combination of something practical, and a Big Picture conviction that grown-ups can be in charge and can be protective. There was something the environment could do and there was something that Jamie could do.

Oliver: I have to completely disagree with what Jamie said. The thing is, he said that our army is protecting us. Guess what, they're only in Iraq. It may not help you much, but I just close my eyes and pretend that the walls and ceiling are full of gorgons. If you look at them, you turn to stone. It helps me fall asleep. I'm not sure if you're such a sci-fi monster lover as I am, but I find that the only opportunity that I have to watch them is at night. A big monster stomping through the streets of Tokyo, stomping on citizens. It's really only special effects or a puppet. It's all fake and none of it really happened. I know you heard about "The Amityville Horror." It's supposed to have really happened. The family who lived in that house announced a few years after the book came out that it was all fake.

GD: He was trying to minimize.

Leo: I used to have that same problem. I used to think about giants when I was little. I solved it by convincing myself that I was immortal. Now I don't worry about death anymore. I got so used to thinking that I was immortal. Pretend you're asleep. That helps. Tossing and turning only makes things worse

MN: Leo was talking about how he would think about giants when he was little, and then solved his distress by being immortal. Then he gave you his real fear: dying.

GD: He went from fearing dying to pretending that he was asleep. Many children think that's what death is really like.

MN: Sleep is, in some ways, like a small death when the heart rate slows down, your breathing becomes shallower, and your body temperature lowers. You have to relinquish control and that is what is so frightening, especially in the face of experiences like the terrorist attacks and the sniper.

GD: This group brought in death. They could tolerate it, whereas the girls' group ended with anorexia, as a means of self-control.

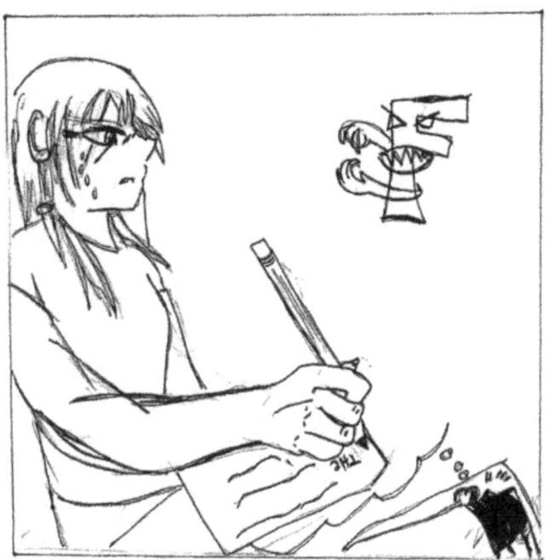

Girls' Group #1

Crystal: I get about four hours of sleep a night. I should probably go to bed earlier. I sleep with my stuffed animals, listen to music and have a night light on. I also read in bed with a clip-on lamp. But one of the things that I do is rock back and forth to go to sleep. I'll show you what it looks like. (She lay on floor and rocked side-to-side). My mom is sick of me doing this because the bed makes so much noise. I also bounce up and down and that moves the bed back and forth. What I do is put the mattress on the floor but my Dad is sick of me doing that. Mom thinks the rocking is bizarre.

GD: Crystal was trying not only to self-regulate when she would get agitated, soothing herself by rocking, but her comment and behavior right then also reflected her response to trauma and neglect. Crystal was in an orphanage in Russia for the first three years of her life. She slept in a communal bed. For her, sleep was hardly restful.

MN: In addition to the regulatory issue that she was describing, she was depicting a body memory of distress.

Abby: I use a night-light but I still can't sleep.

GD: As Abby tried to say this she was holding her breath.

Crystal: I usually wake up at four in the morning and get ice cream. That's when my dad gets up to go to work.

Mallory: What works for me is I make up a story in my head.

Crystal: I hold my guinea pig and think of the day. I also listen to music.

GD: This group's responses to the letter were quite different from the other groups' and reflected the level at which these girls functioned. They struggled day-to-day with problems of self-soothing and coping with anxiety. So it is not surprising that their responses were concrete.

Activities

1. Ask each child to draw or write out a dream that he or she had.
2. Ask children to tell what makes them feel fearful?
   a. Being alone
   b. Being in a new or unfamiliar situation
   c. Being in the dark
   d. Worrying that someone might criticize them or dislike them.
   e. Believing that they will fail.
3. Ask children to describe a time that they felt fearful. Then ask them to show what it looks like in their body when they are scared. How would they talk or move at such times? Then ask children to tell how they make themselves feel safe when they are afraid. Has anyone in the group overcome a fear? How did they do it?
4. Draw a safe place that you can go to when you are worried or afraid. Who helps you to feel safe and secure? Who do you talk to when you are afraid?

References

Annunziata, J., & Nemiroff, M. (2009). *Sometimes I'm scared.* Washington, DC: Magination Press.

Brooks, B., & Siegel, P. M. (1996). *The scared child: Helping kids overcome traumatic events.* New York: Wiley.

DeGangi, G. A., & Kendall, A. (2008). *Effective parenting for the hard-to-manage child.* New York: Routledge.

Rapoport, J. L. (1989). *Obsessive-compulsive disorder in children and adolescents.* Washington, DC: American Psychiatric Press.

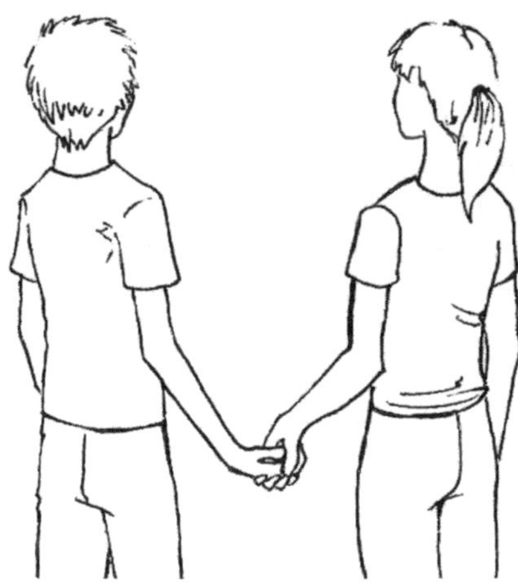